T0291976

Red Flags II: A Guide to Solving Serious Pathology of the Spine

Commissioning Editor: Rita Demetriou-Swanwick
Development Editor: Veronika Watkins, Natalie Meylan
Project Manager: Emma Riley, Vijayakumar Sekar
Designer: George Ajayi
Illustration Manager: Gillian Richards
Illustrator: Jonathan Haste

Red Flags II: A Guide to Solving Serious Pathology of the Spine

Sue Greenhalgh MA, GD Phys, FCSP

Consultant Physiotherapist, Bolton PCT, Bolton, UK
*Honorary Senior Lecturer, School of Public Health and Clinical
Sciences, University of Central Lancashire, Preston, UK*
Fellow of Chartered Society of Physiotherapy, London, England

James Selfe PhD, MA, GD Phys, FCSP

*Professor of Physiotherapy, School of Public Health & Clinical
Sciences, University of Central Lancashire, Preston, UK*
*Fellow of the Chartered Society of Physiotherapy; Visiting
Academic in Physiotherapy Studies, Satakunta Applied
University, Pori, Finland*

Foreword by

Professor Ann Moore
PhD, GradDipPhys, FCSP, DipTP, CertEd, FMACP

ILTM Professor of Physiotherapy, University of Brighton, UK

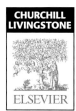

CHURCHILL LIVINGSTONE

ELSEVIER

EDINBURGH   LONDON   NEW YORK
OXFORD   PHILADELPHIA   ST LOUIS
SYDNEY   TORONTO   2010

CHURCHILL
LIVINGSTONE
ELSEVIER

ISBN: 978-0-4430-6914-7

British Library Cataloguing in Publication Data
A catalogue record for this book is available from the British Library

Library of Congress Cataloging in Publication Data
A catalog record for this book is available from the Library of Congress

Note
Knowledge and best practice in this field are constantly changing. As new research and experience broaden our knowledge, changes in practice, treatment and drug therapy may become necessary or appropriate. Readers are advised to check the most current information provided (i) on procedures featured or (ii) by the manufacturer of each product to be administered, to verify the recommended dose or formula, the method and duration of administration, and contraindications. It is the responsibility of the practitioner, relying on their own experience and knowledge of the patient, to make diagnoses, to determine dosages and the best treatment for each individual patient, and to take all appropriate safety precautions. To the fullest extent of the law, neither the Publisher nor the Authors assumes any liability for any injury and/or damage to persons or property arising out of or related to any use of the material contained in this book. It is the responsibility of the treating practitioner, relying on independent expertise and knowledge of the patient, to determine the best treatment and method of application for the patient.

The Publisher

ELSEVIER your source for books,
journals and multimedia
in the health sciences
www.elsevierhealth.com

Working together to grow
libraries in developing countries
www.elsevier.com | www.bookaid.org | www.sabre.org

ELSEVIER BOOK AID International Sabre Foundation

The
publisher's
policy is to use
**paper manufactured
from sustainable forests**

Printed in China

Contents

Foreword

This book significantly builds on the authors' previous text (Greenhalgh S, Selfe J 2006 *Red Flags: a guide to identifying serious pathology of the spine*, Churchill Livingstone, Elsevier, Edinburgh).

The roles of extended scope (advanced practitioners) and consultant physiotherapists in the field of musculoskeletal therapy in medicine have grown exponentially in the past 5 years, with many being first contact practitioners in hospital orthopaedic outpatient settings. These practitioners work with considerable and sometimes complete autonomy. With increasing autonomy comes of course more responsibility, and in the field of spinal pathology accurate differential diagnosis and well-grounded clinical reasoning are essential. Greenhalgh and Selfe have focused wisely in the areas of spinal pathology that present significant challenges to all practitioners who are dealing with patients with these problems on a daily basis.

Although advanced practitioners and consultant physiotherapists have important roles in differential diagnosis on the frontline of musculoskeletal

assessment, all physiotherapists, osteopaths and chiro-
practors, as well as members of the medical profession,
have a duty to recognize Red Flags in the context of
their practice. This text is well placed to fulfil the information needs of all these practitioners dealing with
spinal conditions.

The text usefully includes a section on clinical reasoning which embraces both theoretical and philosoph-
ical standpoints and gives useful examples of reasoning
in the exposition. The evidence base for Red Flags is
addressed in the next chapter which provides the existing evidence that physiotherapists are generally capable
of correctly identifying Red Flags and ensuring the right
management strategy is undertaken. This chapter also
discusses the use of Red Flags as a clinical prediction
guide.

Four chapters in the text are devoted to serious
pathologies: extrapulmonary spinal tuberculosis, cauda
equina syndrome, cancer and serious pathology fractures. Each chapter commences with case descriptions,
and as the chapter proceeds, the reader is challenged
by prompts to guide their reasoning and diagnostic
processes. The chapters also usefully highlight possible
treatments and prognoses of the conditions identified,
having first listed possible Red Herrings and gold
standard investigations.

Chapter 7 focuses on red herrings using clinical
cases and again uses prompts to stimulate the readers'
thought and reasoning processes. Finally, Chapter 8,
which is jointly authored with Andrew Maskell,
Consultant Orthopaedic Surgeon, focuses extremely

well on investigations that may be used to determine the presence and nature of serious pathology of the spine.

The authors are to be congratulated on producing such a useful and thought-provoking text. The information presented here is a vital addition to the musculoskeletal clinician's knowledge base and will, if consumed by those in this field of practice, significantly contribute to the outcomes of patient care.

The book is written in a very user-friendly way while at the same time presenting a series of intellectual challenges mirroring what should happen in everyday practice. As such it provides an exemplar for those just beginning in practice, and also perhaps as a leveller for some clinicians whose knowledge of serious pathology of the spine should be greater. In either case the book can contribute to learning in everyday practice and may highlight the need for further professional development. To clinicians I would say 'Enjoy the read! Celebrate the challenges the book offers you', and to the authors I would say 'Thank you for producing such a well-grounded and informative text'.

Professor Ann P Moore

Acknowledgements

We would like to thank all of the staff from the musculoskeletal service in Bolton Primary Care Trust who contributed to these case studies along with Celia Gardner for the inspiration which has led to this book.

Introduction

This book is intended to help clinicians consider the holistic presentation of the patient. One of the problems we face in this field is the dearth of high-quality evidence. One reason for this is the relatively small numbers of patients involved, as less than 1% of patients with back pain who present to clinicians have serious spinal pathology (Clinical Standards Advisory Group (CSAG) 1994). A lot of the evidence that is available has been developed from clinical observation rather than from scientific study. Traditionally, it is this reflective observational process that has enabled diagnostic processes to be developed. Pattern recognition then enhances clinical practice by increasing the speed of diagnosis. For example, Maitland, McKenzie and Cyriax developed new concepts in approaching musculoskeletal medicine using systems of careful reflective clinical observation. Their individual clinical reasoning processes and pattern recognition enabled them to develop whole systems of assessment and treatment.

Another limitation is that some of the better-quality studies focus narrowly on one or two Red Flags to support the identification of serious spinal pathology. Although this approach may be methodologically robust from a research perspective, this reductionist approach is removed from the real world of clinical practice on a day-to-day basis. Historically, medical diagnosis is based on the combination of thorough history and physical examination. Together these two aspects provide the basic information that the clinician synthesizes to build a picture of the patient's complete problem.

This book will help in approaching the patient with a discriminatory and systematic methodology. We feel that it is important to approach the patient in a logical manner reflecting continuously on the information gathered during the consultation to take the clinician to the next stage of the journey. Using a reflective clinical reasoning process is analogous to reading a map – on a regular basis the reader stops and checks where they are avoiding getting lost. The road map also guides you through the Red Herrings, which could take the clinician down a 'misattribution cul-de-sac'. As clinicians we must all be vigilant and responsive to the relevant signs that are available (Fig. I.1)

The first stage of the journey begins with diagnostic triage.

DIAGNOSTIC TRIAGE (CSAG 1994)

- Simple backache (95% of cases)
- Nerve root pain (<5% of cases)
- Serious spinal pathology (<1% of cases).

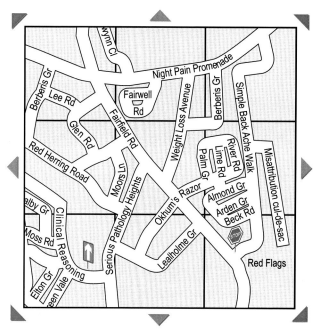

Fig. I.1 The Red Flags street map.

Although such patients are relatively rare, it is well recognized that the earlier patients with serious pathology are identified the better the patient outcome (Wiesel et al 1996). Diagnostic triage is vital as there is little to be gained by requesting a plethora of tests or instigating myriad treatment options unless these have been specifically indicated by the patient's presentation to confirm a particular diagnosis or have been reasoned as appropriate to the presenting condition.

It will not come as a surprise that we have updated the list of Red Flags; we have previously demonstrated how Red Flag lists evolve through time as medicine and the health of populations change (Greenhalgh & Selfe 2006).

UPDATED HIERARCHICAL LIST OF RED FLAGS

- Age >50 years + history of cancer + unexplained weight loss + failure to improve after 1 month of evidence-based conservative therapy

- Age <10 and >51 years
- Medical history (current or past) of:
  - Cancer
  - Tuberculosis
  - Human immunodeficiency virus (HIV)/acquired immune deficiency syndrome (AIDS) or intravenous drug use
  - Osteoporosis
- Weight loss >10% body weight (3–6 months)
- Severe night pain precluding sleep
- Loss of sphincter tone and altered S4 sensation
- Bladder retention or bowel incontinence
- Positive extensor plantar response

- Age 11–19
- Weight loss 5–10% body weight (3–6 months)

- Constant progressive pain
- Band-like pain
- Abdominal pain and changed bowel habits, but with no change of medication
- Inability to lie supine
- Bizarre neurological deficit
- Spasm
- Disturbed gait

🚩

- Loss of mobility, difficulty with stairs, falls, trips
- Legs misbehave, odd feelings in legs, legs feeling heavy
- Weight loss <5% body weight (3–6 months)
- Smoking
- Systemically unwell
- Trauma
- Bilateral pins and needles in hands and/or feet
- Previous failed treatment
- Thoracic pain
- Headache
- Physical appearance
- Marked partial articular restriction of movement

RED HERRINGS

🐟 Misattribution by:

- Patient
- Referring doctor or allied health professional
- Treating physiotherapist

🐟 Inappropriate overt illness behaviour

🐟 Widespread pain systems dysfunction

- ➤ Other conditions that complicate the clinical scenario but which do not impact on the management of the patient
- ➤ Biomedical masqueraders

Internationally, health services are increasingly faced with the need to ensure that professionals provide the most appropriate and timely care to patients. In 2003 New Zealand's Health Workforce Advisory Committee made the following statements:

> 'Simply doing more of the same is not an option'
> 'A major culture change (or paradigm shift) is required'
> 'Some totally new roles and ways of working will emerge'

In the UK, recent developments, such as the New Deal for junior doctors and the European Working Time Directive, have reduced working time for junior medical staff (Health Care Workforce NHS UK 2008). These challenges to healthcare have been met by efforts to change whole systems in order to modernize services. This has included the specific focus on reconsidering the roles of non-medical members of the healthcare team. There has been an increasing drive towards the development of a 'flexible' workforce, where different professionals are able to take on each other's traditional tasks (Table I.1). As a result the UK National Health Service (NHS) has seen the creation of a host of new roles, including extended scope practitioners (McPherson et al 2006).

Table I.1 Classification of changes in skill mix in healthcare (Sibbald et al 2004)

Changing roles	
Enhancement	Increasing the depth of a job by extending the role or skills of a particular group of workers
Substitution	Expanding the breadth of a job, in particular by working across professional divides or exchanging one type of worker for another
Delegation	Moving a task up or down a traditional uni-disciplinary ladder
Innovation	Creating new jobs by introducing a new type of worker
Changing the interface between services	
Transfer	Moving the provision of a service from one healthcare setting to another
Relocation	Shifting the venue from which a service is provided from one healthcare sector to another without changing the people who provide it
Liaison	Using specialists in one healthcare sector to educate and support staff working in another

Part of the whole systems change has stimulated the growth of services such as the Clinical Assessment, Treatment and Support (CATS) service in the NHS, which has developed in recognition of the need to improve the interface between primary and secondary care. CATS services provide an environment in which patients can undergo assessment, diagnosis and treatment in an alternative setting to that of existing hospital outpatient services (McPherson et al 2006). Most of the case histories we present in this book are from anonymized patients presenting to CATS services.

It is clear that traditional models of physiotherapy practice are being significantly challenged by many of the proposed reforms occurring in health services internationally (Nicolls & Larmer 2005). For example, a situation has arisen where physiotherapy practitioners are now increasingly autonomous and taking on new and expanded roles in a wide variety of primary care environments in both public and private sectors. This has important implications for practice; Levack et al (2002) reported that in 23% (n = 72) of their patients, a diagnosis of metastatic cord compression was the first presenting symptom of malignancy. The authors highlighted that in most patients, symptoms started when they were leading normal lives in the community. Patients with serious spinal pathology will most often first present with problems to a clinician in a primary care setting; it is therefore imperative that primary care clinicians, whether employed in the public or private sectors, wherever they are practising, are prepared for this scenario, ask the relevant questions and, where indicated, initiate appropriate further investigations.

In the USA, the majority of physical therapists hold all the privileges associated with autonomous practice, including direct access to physical therapy services, according to the American Physical Therapy Association (APTA Board 2001):

'Autonomous physical therapist practice is practice characterized by independent, self-determined, professional judgment and action. An autonomous physical therapist practitioner, within the scope of practice defined by the Guide to Physical Therapist Practice, *provides physical therapy services to patients/clients who have direct and unrestricted access to their services, and may refer as appropriate to other health care providers and other professionals and for diagnostic tests.'*

In the UK, *Charting the Future*, a position paper (Chartered Society of Physiotherapy (CSP) 2008), is currently under discussion. Some examples of the expectations of members' practice, which may be included, are to:

- Cope with uncertainty
- Make decisions effectively where there is no single 'correct' answer
- Take responsibility for their decisions and be accountable for their actions
- Apply a robust evidence base to their practice, being reflective and thinking critically
- Identify and take responsibility for their own learning and development needs.

Although some practitioners question the appropriateness of autonomous practice, extended roles and shifting of professional boundaries, these changes are unlikely to be reversed, and it can be seen from these examples that both in the USA and the UK, professional bodies have responded by providing professional frameworks that allow flexibility for those who are taking on these new and extended roles.

Finally we would like to use this opportunity to point out a few things about this book. First, all of the case histories are based on actual cases histories of real people; apart from changing the names and any other obvious identifying features, we have tried to present the cases as closely as possible to how they presented to the various clinicians who were involved in their management. This approach does have the disadvantage of leaving some gaps in information and 'rough edges', however, we have deliberately taken this approach to maximize the clinical usefulness of these cases as aids to learning.

Second, it is important to note that the results of biochemical tests vary slightly between different pathology departments. We have tried where possible to quote the normal range as reported by the specific department that conducted the test. This has led to slightly different ranges being quoted and slightly different formats being presented. This is perhaps not as tidy and as consistent as we would have liked to have presented in a book, but once again it does match the real world of clinical practice, where clinicians may have to interpret test results from different pathology departments.

Finally we would like to remind you of one of our favourite quotes:

> 'The identification of serious pathology depends on awareness, vigilance and suspicion rather than a set of rules.'
>
> (Grieve 1994)

References

APTA Board 2001 Definition of autonomous practice. PT Bulletin online 2: no. 11

CSAG 1994 Report of a Clinical Standards Advisory Group on back pain. Her Majesty's Stationery Office, London

CSP 2008 Charting the future of physiotherapy – a position paper. CSP, London

Greenhalgh S, Selfe J 2006 Red flags: a guide to identifying serious pathology of the spine, 1st edn. Churchill Livingstone, Edinburgh

Grieve G P 1994 The masqueraders. In: Boyling J D, Palastanga N (eds) Grieve's modern manual therapy: the vertebral column, 2nd edn. Churchill Livingstone, Edinburgh, pp 841–856

Health Care Workforce NHS UK 2008 Working time directive FAQs. Online. Available: www.healthcareworkforce.nhs.uk/ working_time_directive/general/working_time_directive_ faqs.html (accessed 16 July 2008)

Health Workforce Advisory Committee 2003 The New Zealand health workforce. Future directions – recommendations to the minister of health. Health Workforce Advisory Committee, Wellington

Levack P, Graham J, Collie D et al 2002 Don't wait for a sensory level – listen to the symptoms: a prospective audit of the delays in diagnosis of malignant cord compression. Clinical Oncology 14: 472–480

McPherson K, Kersten K, George S et al 2006 A systematic review of evidence about extended roles for allied health profesionals. Journal of Health Service Research Policy 11: 240–247

Nicolls D, Larmer P 2005 Possible futures for physiotherapy: an exploration of the New Zealand context. New Zealand Journal of Physiotherapy 33: 55–60

Sibbald B, Shen J, McBride A 2004 Changing the skill-mix of the health care workforce. Journal of Health Services Research and Policy 9: 28–38

Wiesel S W, Weinstein J N, Herkowitz H et al 1996 The lumbar spine, 2nd edn. International Society for the Study of the Lumbar Spine, W B Saunders, Philadelphia

Chapter 1

Clinical Reasoning

According to Waddell (2004) up to 40% of back pain patients fear they have some serious disease. This creates an environment in which it could be very easy to be misled. Although this is an important issue, the clinical findings and the clinical reasoning of the clinician must influence the direction of travel. The following extract from a patient's story published in the *BMJ* (Greenway 1994) illustrates this concern over serious pathology very well, especially considering that the patient in question was himself a general practitioner (GP). The patient presented with low back and leg pain. Following a number of consultations with a variety of professionals including a physiotherapist, he sought the help of a neurosurgeon. The surgeon indicated that the signs were not clear-cut, and this caused the patient some alarm!

> *'What did he think it was? Probably a disc but we need to think about ankylosing spondylitis, he said. Unsaid, he must have been thinking of spinal tumours, lymphoma, tuberculosis because I certainly was. For the*

*next week I woke in the early hours thinking I would be
brave and dignified as I approached death. I feared the
ankylosing spondylitis most. I began to grieve the loss
of my love of mountain walking and dinghy sailing. I
tried unsuccessfully to keep my worries from my
partner. She was supportive. We planned for a life of
disability.'*

Clearly this patient's medical background served to
considerably heighten anxiety levels in the face of
clinical uncertainty. As stated in the introduction, as
practitioners we are obliged to accept some degree of
uncertainty during the clinical reasoning process, but
we should remember that this uncertainty could have a
profound effect on the patient if it is visible to them.

Figure 1.1 illustrates varying degrees of certainty
with respect to the theft of a handbag. The index of suspicion is different in response to the different presenta-
tions of the scene of the crime. This logical reasoning
process is synonymous with the clinical reasoning that
takes place in practice.

HISTORICAL PERSPECTIVE

The Hippocratic Oath was written in about 400BC.
Hippocrates was the most prominent physician of
antiquity, and Hippocratic medicine represents the most
significant historical landmark for the evolution of
Western medicine. Before Hippocrates, medicine was
practised as an empirical art that was overtly religious
and superstitious in nature. A modern version of the

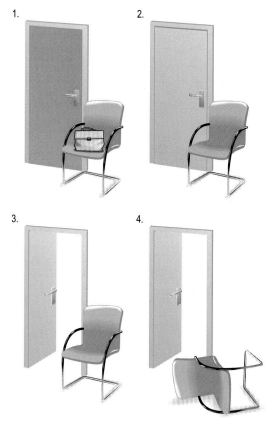

Fig. 1.1 1. Room with handbag, door closed. 2. Room with no handbag, door closed. 3. Room with no handbag, door open. 4. Room with no handbag, door open and room dishevelled.

Hippocratic Oath (Box 1.1, italics added for emphasis) was written in 1964 by Louis Lasagna, Academic Dean of the School of Medicine at Tufts University, USA. This modern version is used in many medical schools around the world today. We have emphasized (text in italics) two of the sections that are particularly relevant to the holistic nature of clinical practice associated with serious spinal pathology.

The Hippocratic approach to medicine assimilated the accumulated knowledge of the past and formed a logical and rational diagnostic system. This was based on a careful, systematic and holistic clinical observation of the individual patient; quintessentially that is exactly what clinicians today should be doing. Hippocrates believed in the healing power of nature and diseases were attributed to natural rather than supernatural causes. It is also interesting to note that Hippocrates treated patients holistically as 'psychosomatic entities' in relation to their natural environment (Marketos & Skiadas 1999) and that he began to document a patient's pallor, pulse, excretion, etc., which are the seeds of a medical subjective history that we would gather in clinical practice today.

Aristotle in the third century BC also made major contributions to medicine, but it is his contribution to clinical reasoning that we wish to focus on here. Aristotlean philosophy used a system of 'practical reasoning' which is still relevant today when considering the possible tension that exists between individual, holistic patient-centred care and the application of evidence-based practice (Gillies & Sheehan 2002). The

Box 1.1 Hippocratic Oath – the modern version (Lasagna 1964)

'I swear to fulfill, to the best of my ability and judgment, this covenant. I will respect the hard-won scientific gains of those physicians in whose steps I walk, and gladly share such knowledge as is mine with those who are to follow. I will apply, for the benefit of the sick, all measures [that] are required, *avoiding those twin traps of overtreatment and therapeutic nihilism. I will remember that there is art to medicine as well as science, and that warmth, sympathy, and understanding may outweigh the surgeon's knife or the chemist's drug. I will not be ashamed to say "I know not," nor will I fail to call in my colleagues when the skills of another are needed for a patient's recovery.* I will respect the privacy of my patients, for their problems are not disclosed to me that the world may know. Most especially must I tread with care in matters of life and death. If it is given me to save a life, all thanks. But it may also be within my power to take a life; this awesome responsibility must be faced with great humbleness and awareness of my own frailty. Above all, I must not play at God. *I will remember that I do not treat a fever chart, a cancerous growth, but a sick human being, whose illness may affect the person's family and economic stability. My responsibility includes these related problems, if I am to care adequately for the sick.* I will prevent disease whenever I can, for prevention is preferable to cure. I will remember that I remain a member of society, with special obligations to all my fellow human beings, those sound of mind and body as well as the infirm. If I do not violate this oath, may I enjoy life and art, respected while I live and remembered with affection thereafter. May I always act so as to preserve the finest traditions of my calling and may I long experience the joy of healing those who seek my help.'

potential problem is that evidence-based practice is developed from populations rather than from individual patients. Clinicians, however, usually see only individual patients at any one time; this leads to the problem that is posed by the question 'What should we do when the individual patient varies from the description of the population on which the best evidence is based?' In addition, the problem of applying robust clinical reasoning in this field of practice is further compounded by the fact that much of the evidence within the Red Flag literature is of a low level.

Gillies & Sheehan's 2002 paper offers a comprehensive and very useful insight into applying Aristotlean philosophy to patient care in the twenty-first century. They focus on **Aristotle's 'practical reasoning'** approach which is a form of clinical decision making that allows for flexibility depending on 'what suits the occasion'. However, they stress that this is not an excuse for careless or sloppy thinking, rather it is an acknowledgement that guidelines can only be based on what has occurred previously. New clinical situations contain many indeterminate elements, some of which may be subtle and ill defined, and unique to that particular situation. Each patient is different and deserves individual consideration, and not an unthinking, automated and crude application of evidence-based practice. Making good clinical decisions is therefore based on making the individuality of the situation central to the process. It is important to stress that this does not imply that evidence-based practice and guidelines have no place in clinical practice; their place is vital to aid accurate decision making when the patient presents with features that suggest their application is appropriate. In summary, Gillies & Sheehan (2002) argue that clinical decision making is the result of a perception by the practitioner of the individual situation that takes into account all of the particulars and not only those that are easily measurable.

Dawes et al (2005) argue that knowledge is either tacit or explicit. Tacit knowledge is non-research knowledge, for example the ability of the healthcare professional to recognize when a patient is ill by their appearance, behaviour and overt symptoms, i.e. 'the wisdom of experience'. Explicit knowledge is based on research evidence. John, who had malignant myeloma, provides a good illustration of this (Greenhalgh & Selfe 2003):

> 'He moved to a chair in reception and sat down and soon began to half lie on to the next chair. Within two minutes he stood up and leaned against a cupboard.'

The department receptionist was tacitly able to recognize the very high level of John's discomfort. Her description to the clinician was then supplemented by explicit knowledge based on specific signs identified during the course of the subjective and objective examination.

To successfully achieve the effective integration of tacit and explicit knowledge in a practical reasoning approach requires well-developed perceptual capacity for 'situational appreciation' and confidence to deal with **indeterminacy**; these qualities develop through training and experience, and require regular, thoughtful reflection on clinical practice.

It is comforting to remember that as clinicians we do not necessarily need to understand complex theories of decision making, however, for those interested in this subject, the next section of this chapter goes on to discuss some of these theories. Finally, before leaving Aristotle it is worth considering his *Categories* – these are individual words and include the following (The Internet Encyclopaedia of Philosophy 2008):

- Quantity
- Quality
- Relation
- Place
- Time
- Situation
- Condition
- Action

Aristotle used these words in this order to 'gain knowledge of an object'. It is interesting to note that if we were asking a patient questions related to the World Health Organization (WHO 2001) International Classification of Function (ICF) components of change in body structures/functions or activities/participation, we could more or less use the same set of words in the same order, and that would give us a large quantity of clinically useful information.

CLINICAL DECISION MAKING

Much of the literature on clinical decision making explores the differences between experts and novices in their approach to problems. Novices tend to rely on abstract principles and piecemeal understanding in contrast with experts, who rely on past experience and holistic understanding (Benner et al 1999). Experts are therefore better able to see the bigger picture of a patient's problem and assess the importance of the combined interaction between many signs and symptoms rather than focusing too narrowly on specific individual items. During this chapter we focus on the idea of the 'big picture' and concentrate on a holistic approach.

A review of the diagnostic accuracy of the subjective history, the objective examination and the erythrocyte sedimentation rate (ESR) in low back pain (van den Hoogen et al 1995) reported that few studies presented data on the diagnostic accuracy of combined positive findings. The authors highlighted this as a problem, as traditionally diagnosis is based on a combination of findings. We have previously discussed the complexity of clinical reasoning processes in serious spinal pathology (Greenhalgh & Selfe 2006). Broadly speaking, models of clinical reasoning are split into two groups:

- Analytic/reductionist
- Holistic/constructionist

Analytic models of clinical decision making as listed by Rashotte & Carnevale (2004) are:

- Bayesian probability (Fischoff & Beyth-Marom 1988)
- Clinical continuum (Hamm 1988)
- Decision analysis (Doubilet & Mcneil 1988)
- Brunswick lens (Wigton et al 1988)
- Information processing (Elstein & Bordage 1988)
- Reflection in action (Schon 1988)

In contrast to these analytic models is a constructionist model in which **intuition** plays a central role. Intuition has not gained legitimacy as an approach to clinical practice (Rashotte & Carnevale 2004) and it is viewed as a basis for irrational acts of guessing (Benner et al 1999). However, intuition and Aristotlean practical reasoning are both of importance to physiotherapy practice and should not be discounted as valid approaches to practice. There is a sound body of evidence supporting the legitimacy of intuition in clinical decision making (Benner et al 1999; Schon 1983; Schon 1988).

Physiotherapy as a profession has problems with both knowledge and evidence. As the physiotherapy paradigm is still emerging from the medical empiricist domination of the past century, physiotherapy knowledge tends to be undervalued. In addition, many routine clinical procedures are not well supported by a strong evidence base (Straszecka 2006). In this chapter, it is the constructionist (holistic) model of clinical reasoning that incorporates intuition and practical reasoning on which we will focus with respect to serious spinal pathology.

Rashotte & Carnevale (2004) identify the following elements of a successful constructionist approach:

- Recognition that each case is unique
- Identification of elements that are familiar and unfamiliar
- Conduct 'on-the-spot' experimentation for competing hypotheses
- Maintain openness to revising opinions

In our previous model of three-dimensional (3D) thinking, we proposed that during patient consultations, a physiotherapist draws on their previous experience and knowledge, and that, simultaneously, each patient consultation adds to the physiotherapist's knowledge and experience. Developing this model further (Fig. 1.2), it is important to note that during a patient consultation each new piece of information gained by the therapist is assessed for diagnostic alternatives – each of which is simultaneously assigned with levels of **certainty** and **plausibility** by the therapist.

Plausibility will be derived mainly from the therapist's previous experience; certainty will be derived mainly from the therapist's existing knowledge base. On completion of the initial assessment, a hierarchy of diagnostic hypotheses is compiled by the therapist and a diagnostic conclusion reached, which is referred to as 'the conclusion of the greatest belief' (Straszecka 2006) (Fig. 1.3). The conclusion of the greatest belief then informs the decision making of the therapist in terms of informing the next stage of the patient's journey. For

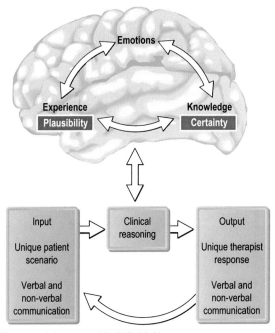

Fig. 1.2   Adapted model of 3D thinking.

example, in some complex situations it may be extremely difficult to interpret non-classic signs and symptoms, therefore the clinician's conclusion of greatest belief will suggest that further diagnostic testing or onward refer-ral to a specialist is indicated. Using this kind of termi-nology is very useful as it helps to remind us that we

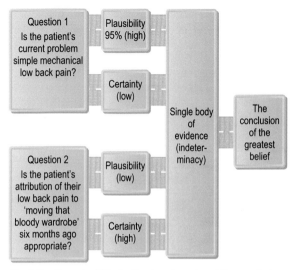

Fig. 1.3 Flow chart illustrating how to arrive at the conclusion of the greatest belief.

work with uncertainty and imprecision in our clinical decision making on a day-to-day basis, and that what we are actually doing is generating hypotheses.

One of the reasons for uncertainty in any clinical encounter is that the cause and subsequent course of any specific disease or condition is idiosyncratic, i.e. heterogeneous disease presentation. Put more simply, the same disease or condition will manifest itself differently in different people at different times. This is a key challenge for therapists and one which we attempt to address in this book by using multiple real patient case histories. Similarly clinicians working across different boundaries and timelines of a disease will have a different perspective of that disease process. Another important aspect of uncertainty stems from indeterminacy, which is present within any system of clinical reasoning. Indeterminacy arises from the reality that the patient cannot possibly, and sometimes does not, tell the therapist everything that may be relevant to their current condition.

Many patients have no underlying medical knowledge and so are in a position of ignorance as to what may be clinically important. Sometimes, as in the case of the GP we discussed earlier, those who do have training are no better off than those without. Most patients are not able to offer the relevant information to assist the clinician in decision making without the relevant prompts. A good example of this is the case of Margaret, who did not tell the therapist about the lump in her breast (Greenhalgh & Selfe 2004). Therapists themselves also contribute to indeterminacy, as a therapist cannot possibly know everything that may be relevant to the current condition. The combination of patient and therapist factors leads to a greater or lesser degree of indeterminacy for every patient. Therapists need to proceed along a journey of discovery, establishing levels of plausibility and certainty by extracting the relevant information with appropriate prompts. When considering the nature of evidence during the implementation of evidence-based practice it is important to remember that traditionally in statistical theory, any evidence not supporting a hypothesis is considered as evidence for the refutation of the hypothesis; there is no allowance made for Aristotlean practical reasoning, intuition or clinical indeterminacy.

We have previously discussed Bayes' theorem as an aid to diagnosis (Greenhalgh & Selfe 2006). Thomas Bayes was an eighteenth-century mathematician, and his theorem concerns conditional probabilities. According to Chalmers (2003) these are:

'Probabilities for propositions that depend on (and hence are conditional on) the evidence bearing on those propositions.'

Put another way, the probability ascribed to an event depends on prior knowledge of the event, and if any new evidence pertaining to the circumstances of the event come to light, the probability (related to the event) changes in response to the new evidence. The Dempster–Shafer theory, also known as the Theory of Belief Functions, is a generalization of the Bayesian theory of subjective probability (Shafer 2006) and helps to overcome the problem of indeterminacy outlined above. Whereas the Bayesian theory requires probabilities for each question of interest, belief functions allow for degrees of belief for one question based on probabilities for a related question. Shafer (2006) uses the following example as an illustration of how we can obtain degrees of belief for the question:

- Did a tree fall on my car?

from the probabilities of another question:

● Is the witness reliable?

In a more relevant clinical example we can obtain degrees of belief for the important question:

● Is the patient's current problem simple mechanical low back pain?

As we are unable to elicit a direct answer to this specific question we ask:

● Is the patient's attribution of their low back pain to 'moving that bloody wardrobe' six months ago appropriate?

The answer to this second question is assigned with levels of certainty and plausibility, and this, along with *all* the other evidence gained from the assessment, helps to generate the conclusion of the greatest belief (see Fig. 1.3).

Apart from helping to overcome the problem of indeterminacy in clinical practice, another advantage of the Dempster–Shafer theory is that it allows evidence from multiple sources to be combined within the same frame of reference into one body of evidence. This process of combining disparate evidence into a single body of evidence leads, as we have said earlier, to the conclusion of the greatest belief. The conclusion of the greatest belief is very much central to what we are trying to promote when thinking about clinical decision making and Red Flags. It is important that a complete and holistic picture, in line with the biopsychosocial model paradigm of the ICF, of the patient is compiled and that a consideration of the combination of Red Flags feeds directly into a therapist's clinical reasoning, in order to inform the conclusion of the greatest belief.

Key points in this section

- Aristotlean practical reasoning
- Intuition
- Clinical indeterminacy
- The conclusion of the greatest belief

The above are all important elements for understanding the constructionist approach to clinical reasoning that will lead to a holistic picture of the patient's problems.

When you are reading the case histories in this book, and later when you are back in clinic, it may be useful for you to refer occasionally to this page and answer some of the following questions, to help focus your clinical reasoning.

What are you thinking now?
What is your index of suspicion?
How many / are present?
What other flags are present?
What are your diagnostic alternatives?
What is challenging about this case?
What assumptions have you made about this case?
What is your level of plausibility and certainty?
What will you do next with this patient?

What have you learnt from this case?
Will you change your future practice?

INTERNATIONAL CLASSIFICATION OF FUNCTIONING, DISABILITY AND HEALTH (ICF)

Clinicians are constantly being reminded that in order to be a successful practitioner they need to treat the patient from a holistic perspective. Sometimes in the day-to-day management of patients in a busy clinic this may seem like an unrealistic ideal, however the ICF provides a useful and practical framework for clinical practice (Mittrach et al 2008; WHO 2001). The ICF was endorsed by the WHO in 2001, and it presents a holistic biopsychosocial paradigm. According to Mittrach et al (2008) the medical model of health views disability as a problem of the individual, caused by injury or disease. The social model of health defines disability as a lack of integration of an individual into society. The ICF combines these two models by viewing functioning not only in association with morbidity, but also in the interaction with personal factors and the environment. The ICF describes health from the perspective of the body, the individual and the society. The framework is divided into two parts, each with two components. Each component can be expressed in positive or negative terms:

- Part 1: Functioning and Disability
    - Body Functions and Structures
    - Activities and Participation
- Part 2: Contextual Factors
    - Environment
    - Personal

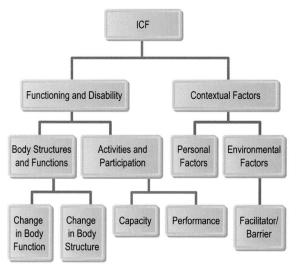

Fig. 1.4 Structure of the International Classification of Functioning, Disability and Health (ICF).

It is useful to visualize the relationship between the various parts of the framework (Fig. 1.4). At first glance the usefulness of such a framework may not seem immediately apparent, however, when considering the complex and multifactorial nature of the serious pathologies that give rise to multiple Red Herrings and

Red Flags, the ICF does have a place in clinical practice. For example, tuberculosis is a disease of poverty associated with poor environmental living conditions. The case of Alice in Chapter 3 provides a good example of when it is highly relevant for clinicians to ask contextual questions about environmental factors.

From a clinical perspective, people will usually notice negative changes in their *Functioning and Disability*; these are often due to changes in *Body Structure or Function*. When these changes are also associated with a reduction in *Capacity and/or Performance*, limitations in *Activity* and *Participation* will manifest themselves. Once the changes in *Functioning and Disability* pass a *Personal* threshold a person may seek medical help. At all stages these processes may be subject to modification by the *Environment* in which the person lives or works. The holistic nature of the ICF is illustrated in Figure 1.5. It is worth noting here that many of the conditions to which we refer in this book have extended prodromal periods where subtle changes in a person's *Body Structure or Function* occur over protracted timescales. These will sometimes manifest themselves as ill-defined symptoms that people are most likely to notice as subtle changes in *Body Function*. One of the case histories we published previously, of John who had a malignant myeloma of the spine, provides a good example of this:

> 'John's problems began 10 months before, in December. His initial symptoms were abdominal pain and increasing problems with constipation despite no changes in

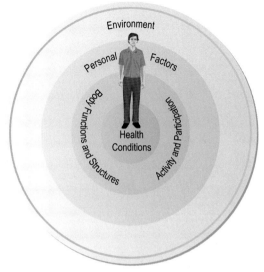

Fig. 1.5 Holistic nature of the International Classification of Functioning, Disability and Health (ICF).

medication. There was no previous history of these symptoms.'

(Greenhalgh & Selfe 2003)

It is imperative that clinicians remain alert to any such indeterminate and sometimes vague reports of changes in body function; other examples include 'feeling out of sorts', 'feeling lethargic/tired' or 'legs feeling heavy/odd'.

THE PRODROMAL PHASE

Gould (2006), in writing specifically about cancer, describes three distinct clinical phases:

- Subclinical – pathological changes but no signs and symptoms
- Prodromal – vague, non-specific symptoms, few if any signs
- Clinical – well-developed signs and symptoms

These three phases are applicable to most major pathologies that present with vague musculoskeletal signs and symptoms (Fig. 1.6).

The prodromal phase of any major pathology is particularly important for primary contact clinicians. During this phase, there tend to be a large number of Red Herrings associated with a high level of clinical

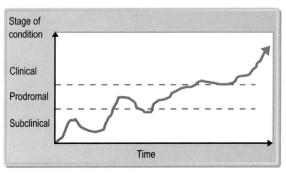

Fig. 1.6 The non-linear course of pathology through subclinical, prodromal and clinical phases.

indeterminacy; this coupled with a low index of suspicion with few if any Red Flags leads to a situation where clinical reasoning can easily become diverted. At this stage the only Red Flag may be age above 50. Once the index of suspicion passes a critical threshold, the therapist will become concerned about the underlying cause of a patient's complaint. The threshold of concern should be set sufficiently low so as not to jeopardize patients' management (Straszecka 2006) (Fig. 1.7), but it should be high enough to not cause unnecessary anxiety and distress. Striking the correct balance between these two factors requires skilful clinical judgement.

It is common that during the prodromal phase, Red Herrings lead to misattribution which can cloud the clinical picture. This is illustrated in Figure 1.8. We have likened the prodromal phase to a tunnel; when the patient enters the tunnel, their journey is continuing but it is very difficult for a clinician to know exactly what is going on. The tunnel also represents the clinical transition from asymptomatic to symptomatic. The river is a reference to Caesar's crossing of the River Rubicon in northern Italy, in 50BC, in his march to Rome, since which time the phrase 'to cross the Rubicon' has meant to pass the point of no return.

In their review, van den Hoogen et al (1995) point out that the role time plays is almost completely ignored in the diagnostic process despite it having the potential to be a valuable diagnostic criterion. Subjective and objective examination in healthy subjects will produce Red Herrings; in a clinical context these would represent chance false-positive findings in patients without

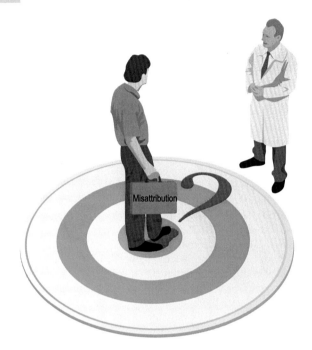

How certain are you?
Where is the threshold for your index of suspicion?

Fig. 1.7 Where is the threshold for your index of suspicion?

disease (Deyo & Hope 2005). It is important to realize that these Red Herrings are often unlikely to be reproducible over time. Constant monitoring and vigilance are therefore crucial in the early stages of benign low

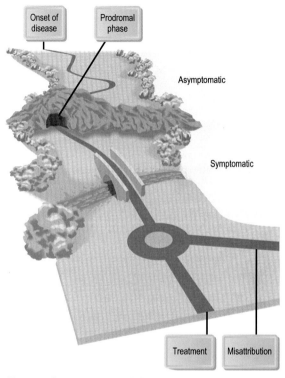

Fig. 1.8 Stages in a patient's journey.

back pain or in the prodromal phase of more serious conditions. It is important for clinicians to understand that the relationship between time and the development of symptoms related to serious pathology is not necessarily linear and that temporary improvements may occur (see Fig. 1.6). This is illustrated very well by the case of Annie in Chapter 5.

Annie's condition was going through a phase of temporary improvement just at the time when she consulted the physiotherapist. She appeared to have responded well to manual treatment and had been compliant with following the advice given to her. These factors significantly influenced the physiotherapist's management of Annie's condition. Although Annie's condition was fairly advanced, it is not unusual during the prodromal phase to find that patients appear to have responded to treatment interventions, often gaining temporary relief at some stage during this phase. This apparent improvement may be due to a complex set of reasons, including, among other things, a placebo response and a willingness to try to please the therapist. However, it is important to realize that any response to treatment tends to be short lived and is superimposed on an underlying worsening trend. A clinician needs to be particularly alert to any changes in the underlying condition and re-evaluate the patient's condition regularly.

Ideally patients should be studied at a uniform time in a disease process to avoid missing important outcomes by starting the clock too late. The optimum time to start a study is at the first clinical manifestation of the disease process (inception cohort) (Straus et al 2005). However, in the real world of clinical practice, patients present to the clinician at different times in the timeline of the disease process with multiple confounding variables. It is interesting to consider whether the disease always becomes symptomatic and presents at the same stage, for example how many cases do we hear about in our career in which the cancer sufferer was unwell for only weeks rather than months? On the other hand, it is very common to observe magnetic resonance imaging (MRI) or X-ray abnormalities which are of no clinical significance (Deyo & Hope 2005).

It is often the case that once a serious pathology has passed the clinical threshold there is a rapid acceleration in the development of the condition with corresponding deterioration in the patient's health. It should be borne in mind that many patients with common cancers are already incurable by the time the disease is diagnosed. This is a very depressing fact; however, clinicians should remember that, generally speaking, the earlier the diagnosis, the greater the survival time. The point at which a cancer has developed sufficiently to become incurable has been termed the 'escape from cure' (Tannock & Hill 1998). This is represented in Figure 1.8, once the bridge over the river has been crossed. However, it would also be true to say that generally the earlier these conditions are diagnosed, the better is the quality of life remaining, because of, for example, better pain control or the preservation of spinal column stability.

IDENTIFYING SERIOUS PATHOLOGY AND THE EMOTIONAL REACTION OF THE CLINICIAN

So far we have tended to discuss the issue of serious pathology in a detached and academic way, although an emotional component is included in the model of 3D thinking (see Fig 1.2). However, the reaction of most clinicians when they realize for the first time that their patient has serious pathology is far from detached. Traditionally, allied health workers have been ill prepared for the emotional turmoil and anxiety experienced when identifying serious spinal pathology. However, with the redesigning of roles, more clinicians are moving into situations where they may indeed be the first person, rather than a doctor, to identify serious pathology. There are two aspects to consider about this position. The first relates to the confidence the clinician has in their own clinical reasoning processes in order to accept that the conclusion of greatest belief is indicating a serious pathology. The second is when serious pathology has been identified. How do they proceed with breaking the bad news to the patient – do they refer the patient to someone else or do they undertake to do this themselves?

During a mentorship session with Judy, an experienced clinician, the following issues were raised with respect to her confidence. At a particular stage of the patient consultation, it became apparent that she was the only person who had enough pieces of the jigsaw of the clinical presentation to realize that the patient had serious pathology. Judy expressed the emotions she felt in the face of this realization while in front of her sat a pleasant, polite elderly man:

'Oh no, not him!'

Suddenly Judy felt that she was working outside her competencies and was engulfed with an almost overwhelming sensation of feeling out of her depth. At this point, the subjective and objective Red Flags, the blood test and imaging results clearly pointed to a conclusion of greatest belief of serious pathology. Judy's interpretation of the examination and results at each stage of the clinical reasoning process was sound and robust. In this case, any of the medical clinicians within the same team would have clinically reasoned in the same way and come to the same conclusion. What then made Judy feel out of her depth? This was the first time that she had experienced the emotional catharsis of being the first to know the situation was serious. This very strong emotion, experienced for the first time, most likely provoked the feeling of being out of her depth. It is easy to assume that doctors will have past experience to draw on in this situation and so for them it is in some way easier to deal with these situations. However, doctors are also likely to have experienced the same turmoil when faced with their first exposure to this situation, despite their medical training. One of our senior medical colleagues asked recently:

'Why do these cases always turn up last thing on a Friday afternoon or the day before I am going on holiday?'

While initially this may appear to be a rather flippant remark about a serious subject, it underlines a key message. That is, even this clinician worries about such cases – they cause him emotional stress and anxiety, spoiling his weekend or holiday, even though he has regularly dealt with them over many years.

The second issue to consider is that of bad news, but first we need to consider what is bad news from a patient's rather than a clinical perspective. Buckman (1992) defines bad news as:

> *'any information, which adversely and seriously affects an individual's view of his or her future.'*

In the context of this book this could be:

- Your pain is unlikely to ever go away
- Your bladder function is unlikely to return
- I suspect that you may have a malignancy

No one likes breaking bad news, so it is important to understand how the delivery of bad news affects patients, their family/carers and clinicians (Taylor 1995). Breaking bad news is a complex communication task that requires expert verbal and non-verbal skills (Department of Health 2003). This complexity can create serious miscommunications, such as a patient misunderstanding the prognosis of their illness or purpose of care (Davis 1991; Hoy 1985). When bad news is delivered poorly, the experience may stay in a patient's or family's mind long after the initial shock of the news has been dealt with. For example, Laura, at the end of a routine check-up, was told by her doctor to make an appointment with the breast cancer nurse. The doctor had incorrectly assumed that Laura had already received her diagnosis, when in fact she did not know she had been diagnosed with breast cancer. The shock and emotional pain of this experience is still felt more strongly by Laura than the suffering she went through during chemotherapy.

Peteet et al (1991) report that patients who are being given bad news want their clinician to be honest, compassionate, caring, hopeful and informative. They also want to be told in person, in a private setting, at their pace, with time for discussion, and, quite often, with a supportive person present.

Being the person responsible for breaking bad news can be extremely stressful for the clinician involved (Department of Health 2003). Evidence suggests that the bearer of bad news experiences strong emotions such as:

- Anxiety
- A burden of responsibility for the news
- Fear of a negative response

This stress can result in a reluctance to deliver bad news (Tesser et al 1971).

It is important to recognize the potential stress that breaking bad news can cause. It is important, for all staff, including senior staff, to reflect on the experience, as appropriate, with their clinical supervisor or mentor as soon as possible after the event (Department of Health 2003). It is also wise to discuss who is responsible for breaking bad news before the event occurs.

Clinicians should be prepared for unpredictable responses to what they consider to be bad news, for instance Ethel in Chapter 6 was actually reassured that something definite had been found to explain her symptoms.

Finally before leaving this subject, it is important to remember that clinicians must also be well prepared for the patient who asks the question:

'Do you think that something is seriously wrong with me?'

We have previously discussed strategies for dealing with this scenario (Greenhalgh & Selfe 2006).

References

Benner P, Hooper-Kyriakidis P, Stannard D 1999 Clinical wisdom and interventions in critical care: a thinking in action approach. W B Saunders, Philadelphia

Buckman R 1992 Breaking bad news: a guide for health care professionals. John Hopkins University Press, Baltimore

Chalmers A F 2003 What is this thing called science? 3rd edn. Open University Press, Maidenhead

Davis H 1991 Breaking bad news. Practitioner 235: 522–526

Dawes M, Summerskill W, Glaziou P et al 2005 Sicily statement on evidence based practice. BMC Medical Education 5: 1

Department of Health, Social Services and Public Safety 2003 Breaking bad news. Department of Health, Social Services and Public Safety, Belfast

Deyo R A, Hope D L 2005 Hope or hype. AMACOM, New York

Doubilet P, Mcneil B J 1988 Clinical decision making. In: Dowie J, Elstein A (eds) Professional judgment: a reader in clinical decision making. Cambridge University Press, Cambridge, pp 255–276

Elstein A, Bordage G 1988 Psychology of clinical reasoning. In: Dowie J, Elstein A (eds) Professional judgment: a reader in clinical decision making. Cambridge University Press, Cambridge, pp 109–129

Fischoff B, Beyth-Marom R 1988 Hypothesis evaluation from a Bayesian perspective. In: Dowie J, Elstein A (eds) Professional judgment: a reader in clinical decision making. Cambridge University Press, Cambridge, pp 323–348

Gillies J, Sheehan M 2002 Practical reasoning and decision making – Hippocrates' problem, Aristotle's answer. British Journal of General Practice 52: 518–519

Gould B E 2006 Pathophysiology for the health professions, 3rd edn. Saunders, Philadelphia

Greenhalgh S, Selfe J 2003 Malignant myeloma of the spine. Physiotherapy 89: 486–488

Greenhalgh S, Selfe J 2004 Margaret: a tragic case of spinal red flags and red herrings. Physiotherapy 90: 73–76

Greenhalgh S, Selfe J 2006 Red flags: a guide to identifying serious pathology of the spine. Churchill Livingstone, Elsevier, Edinburgh

Greenway T 1994 Through uncharted waters. BMJ 308: 143

Hamm R M 1988 Clinical intuition and clinical analysis: expertise and the cognitive continuum. In: Dowie J, Elstein A (eds) Professional judgment: a reader in clinical decision making. Cambridge University Press, Cambridge, pp 78–105

Hoy A M 1985 Breaking bad news to patients. British Journal of Hospital Medicine 34: 96–99

Lasagna L 1964 The hippocratic oath: modern version. Online. Available: www.pbs.org/wgbh/nova/doctors/oath_modern.html (accessed 4 March 2008)

Marketos S G, Skiadas P K 1999 The modern hippocratic tradition: some messages for contemporary medicine. Spine 24: 1159

Mittrach R, Grill E, Walchner-Bonjean M et al 2008 Goals of physiotherapy interventions can be described using the International Classification of Functioning, Disability and Health. Physiotherapy 94: 150–157

Peteet J, Abrams H, Ross D M et al 1991 Presenting a diagnosis of cancer: patients' views. Journal of Family Practice 32: 581

Rashotte J, Carnevale F A 2004 Medical and nursing clinical decision making: a comparative epistemological analysis. Nursing Philosophy 5: 160–174

Schon D A 1983 The reflective practitioner: how professionals think in action. Basic Books, New York

Schon D A 1988 From technical rationality to reflection in action. In: Dowie J, Elstein A (eds) Professional judgment: a reader in clinical decision making. Cambridge University Press, Cambridge, pp 60–77

Shafer G 2006 Dempster–Shafer theory. Online. Available: www.glennshafer.com/assets/downloads/articles/article48. pdf (accessed 4 March 2008)

Straszecka E 2006 Combining uncertainty and imprecision in models of medical diagnosis. Information Sciences 176: 3026–3059

Straus E S, Richardson W S, Glasziou P et al 2005 Evidence-based medicine: how to practice and teach EBM, 3rd edn. Elsevier, Edinburgh

Tannock I F, Hill R P 1998 The basic science of oncology, 3rd edn. McGraw Hill, New York

Taylor S E 1995 Health psychology. McGraw-Hill, New York

Tesser A, Rosen S, Tesser M 1971 On the reluctance to communicate undesirable messages. Psychological Reports 29: 651–654

The Internet Encyclopaedia of Philosophy. Aristotle: a general introduction. Online. Available: www.iep.utm.edu/a/aristotl.htm (accessed 4 March 2008)

van den Hoogen H M, Koes B W, van Eijk J K et al 1995 On the accuracy of history, physical examination, and erythrocyte sedimentation rate in diagnosing low back pain in general practice. A criteria-based review of the literature. Spine 20: 318–327

Waddell G 2004 The back pain revolution, 2nd edn. Churchill Livingstone, Edinburgh

World Health Organization 2001 International Classification of Functioning, Disability and Health. World Health Organization, Geneva

Wigton R S, Hoellerich V L, Patil K D 1988 How physicians use clinical information in diagnosing pulmonary embolism: an application of conjoint analysis. In: Dowie J, Elstein A (eds) Professional judgment: a reader in clinical decision making. Cambridge University Press, Cambridge, pp 130–149

Chapter 2

The Evidence Base for Red Flags

For some years now, the major international guidelines on managing low back pain have been consistent in recommending screening for Red Flags:

- Agency for Health Care Policy and Research (AHCPR; Bigos 1994)
- Clinical Standards Advisory Group (CSAG 1994)
- Royal College of General Practitioners (2001)
- National Institute for Health and Clinical Excellence (NICE 2001)
- European Union (2004)
- New Zealand Ministry of Health (2004)
- Prodigy (2005; now called Clinical Knowledge Summaries)
- Chartered Society of Physiotherapy (CSP 2007)

The recommendations found in these guidelines are also reinforced by many eminent authorities on low back pain, for example Wiesel et al (1996) state:

'It is imperative that characteristics of spinal serious pathology are recognised and acted upon quickly.'

In the light of this, it is interesting to pause and consider what Red Flags actually are.

Red Flags are a list of prognostic variables for serious pathology, i.e.:

- Tumour: benign or malignant
- Infection
- Fracture
- Cauda equina syndrome

Generally, Red Flags have been developed using clinical observation and retrospective analysis. Unfortunately, with a few exceptions, the prognostic strength of individual Red Flags or combinations of Red Flags is not known. To be considered prognostic, a variable need not necessarily be caused by a particular pathological process but it must be strongly associated with the development of a specific outcome in order to predict its occurrence. Demographic variables such as age and gender are often considered prognostic. Risk factors are considered to be distinct from prognostic factors and are often related to lifestyle. For example, smoking is an important risk factor in developing lung cancer, but tumour stage is the most important prognostic factor in individuals who have the disease (Straus et al 2005).

Owing to the way that Red Flag lists have evolved and developed, there is an almost overwhelming profusion of Red Flags. Against this background, it is therefore interesting to consider what evidence there is to support the identification and use of Red Flags in clinical practice.

The recently published clinical guidelines for the physiotherapy management of persistent low back pain (CSP 2007) state that 119 items in the subjective history and 44 items in the objective history have been identified as Red Flags. In addition, these guidelines state that there is wide variation in the definition of a 'Red Flag'. As part of the process, members of the development group were surveyed for levels of agreement on the individual Red Flag items; the results were categorized as follows (Roberts et al 2007):

- 100% agreement = Unanimity
- 75–99% agreement = Consensus
- 51–74% agreement = Majority view
- 0–50% agreement = No consensus

No Red Flag item achieved 100% agreement, however the guidelines reported that the following 11 items were consistently present in more than 50% of the papers reviewed as part of the guideline development process. The level of agreement on the item between the panel members is also presented (CSP 2007; Roberts et al 2007):

- Consensus (level of agreement: 75–99%)
  - Weight loss
  - Previous history of cancer
- Majority view (level of agreement: 51–74%)
  - Night pain
  - Age above 50 years
  - Violent trauma
  - Fever

- Saddle anaesthesia
- Difficulty with micturition
- Intravenous drug misuse
- Progressive neurology
- Systemic steroids

Henschke & Maher (2006) are critical of the evidence supporting Red Flags and argue that there is little primary research in this area and that many guidelines rely on secondary citations. They state:

'there is little or no high-quality evidence on the diagnostic accuracy of red flags and that on the limited evidence available; some red flags seem to have little diagnostic power.'

Klaber-Moffett et al (2006) concur:

'the evidence for red flags is under-developed.'

Chorti (personal communication 2007) conducted a systematic review of Red Flags for spinal malignancies in patients with spinal symptoms and concluded:

- There were few papers published
- Papers often suffered from weak methodology
- Papers were poorly indexed and therefore hard to find

The interest in evidence-based medicine (EBM) has grown since the coining of the phrase in 1991 (Guyatt 1991).

'Evidence based medicine is the conscientious, explicit and judicious use of current best evidence in making decisions about the care of individual patients'

(Sackett et al 1996)

It is important to remember that successful evidence-based practice (EBP) comprises two key components:

High-quality research + sound clinical experience = EBP

EBP is therefore not restricted to randomized trials and meta-analyses; it involves using the best external evidence to answer clinical questions (Sackett et al 1996). EBP therefore requires the complex integration of the best research evidence with clinical expertise when faced with a set of unique patient values and circumstances. Within an evidence-based framework, the research evidence should be valid and clinically relevant. Dawes et al (2005) argue that EBP decisions:

'should be made by those receiving care informed by the tacit and explicit knowledge of those providing care, within the context of available resources.'

When considering Red Flags, we need to think about two dimensions of evidence:

- Evidence that clinicians can successfully identify Red Flags
- Evidence that Red Flags are useful clinical prediction guides

CAN CLINICIANS IDENTIFY RED FLAGS?

A study of 235 primary healthcare physicians and physiotherapists in Sweden (Overmeer et al 2005) reported that 40% of physicians and 25% of physiotherapists were unfamiliar with Red Flags. The authors concluded that a relatively large proportion of clinicians were unfamiliar with the concept of Red Flags. It is interesting that the physiotherapists demonstrated greater Red Flag awareness than the doctors.

In a survey of 1000 physiotherapists in private practice in the USA, 12 paper-based case scenarios were presented to the therapists (Jette et al 2006). Respondents were asked to choose a course of management based on one of three choices:

- Provide physiotherapy intervention to the patient without medical referral
- Provide intervention and then refer the patient to a medical professional
- Refer the patient to a medical professional before any physiotherapy intervention

Three of the 12 scenarios contained significant Red Flags requiring urgent medical attention. Across all cases related to the critical medical conditions, respondents made a correct management decision for 79% of them. For each case individually, 67.6–93.4% made a correct management decision. Nearly 50% of the respondents made a correct management decision for all critical medical cases.

More recently, also in the USA, Leerar et al (2007) reviewed the clinic charts of 160 patients with low back pain, noting the presence or absence of the following 11 Red Flags:

- Age >50
- Bladder dysfunction

- History of cancer
- Immune suppression
- Night pain
- History of trauma
- Saddle anaesthesia
- Lower extremity neurological deficit
- Weight loss
- Recent infection
- Fever/chills

Ninety six per cent of the charts reviewed had at least 64% of the Red Flag items documented. Three items emerged that were not regularly documented: weight loss, recent infection and fever/chills.

Although not extensive, the evidence appears to support the idea that physiotherapists are generally capable of correctly identifying most Red Flags and invoking the appropriate management strategies when faced with Red Flags. However, considering that internationally allied health professional roles are changing and being redefined, giving greater clinical autonomy, it is also clear that there is room for improvement in this area and attention should be paid to increased training opportunities for the identification of Red Flags in both undergraduate and postgraduate curricula.

ARE RED FLAGS USEFUL CLINICAL PREDICTION GUIDES?

Using a qualitative methodology, nominal group technique (NGT) followed by a focus group, we recently investigated whether palliative care clinicians would validate existing Red Flag lists routinely used by clinicians working in primary care (Greenhalgh & Selfe 2008). This approach followed a model proposed by Sibbald et al (2004), in which specialists in one healthcare sector can educate staff working in another. The participants were seven senior palliative care clinicians working at St Catherine's Hospice in northwest England. This group was specifically chosen as we wanted to draw from their experiential knowledge, because palliative care staff have the advantage that once patients are in their care, a definitive diagnosis will have been made. We were interested to hear from the participants about subtle changes that patients reported had occurred in the early stages of their disease. The study explored real stories from patients who were confirmed as having serious spinal pathology.

During the NGT, 37 separate items were generated; 10 items were repeated more than once. The data were subjected to a thematic analysis, which revealed nine separate themes:

- Pain
- Previous history of malignancy
- Neurological deficit
- Bladder and bowel symptoms
- Vague non-specific lower limb symptoms, for example legs feeling heavy
- Failure to respond to standard treatment
- Decreased mobility
- Difficulty breathing
- Absence of previous back pain

The NGT appeared to be a very successful method to generate these data. The participants were fully engaged with the process and a large number of items emerged. Most of the items generated validated well-known items which regularly appear on lists as Red Flags for serious spinal pathology. This finding is reassuring as the study participants were clinicians working exclusively with patients of known diagnosis; it is also worth noting that there was a high degree of agreement in relation to these items. However, three new items emerged, for which there was strong agreement among the participants, and to our knowledge these do not appear on any recognized Red Flag lists used internationally. These items are:

- Band-like trunk pain
- Vague non-specific lower limb symptoms
- Decreased mobility

One week later, we conducted a focus group with the same group of clinicians in order to explore in more detail the themes that had emerged from the NGT, and then to explore in further detail the existing Red Flag lists. Some of the data generated related to the three 'new' Red Flag items are summarized below.

- Band-like trunk pain
  - Often preceded by vague symptoms
  - Commonly bilateral
  - Seems to be related to bone or nerve root
- Vague non-specific lower limb symptoms
  - Common in this group of patients

- Early reported symptom but comes on relatively late in disease progression
- Often pre-dates overt spinal cord compression
- Heaviness preceded by legs feeling odd or strange
- Need to ask 'How do your legs feel?'
- Patients report 'legs misbehave', i.e. will not do what patients want them to do
- May be related to fatigue, muscle weakness, medications or bed rest
- Associated, in particular, with gynaecological cancers
- Decreased mobility
  - May have mild foot drop
  - Leg drags
  - Patients often do not recognize these symptoms as important or significant

Following the work at St Catherine's Hospice, we have started working in collaboration with physiotherapists from Christie Hospital, Manchester, an international oncology centre. This hospital has recently produced a set of guidelines that include a number of items to assist primary care clinicians in the identification of malignant spinal cord compression (MSCC or MCC) (Christie Hospital NHS Foundation Trust 2007):

- Previous diagnosis of cancer
- New spinal pain, particularly thoracic/root pain
- Description of 'tight band around chest' or nerve-like pain in upper thighs

- Significant change in long-standing pain (unremitting, feeling of despair)
- New difficulty in climbing up stairs
- Unsteadiness/heaviness in legs
- Tingling or electric shock in spine with Valsalva manoeuvre, e.g. cough, sneeze, neck flexion

Despite being developed independently, it is interesting to note the high level of agreement between the Christie Hospital list and the list of items generated at St Catherine's Hospice. Some of these items appear to be worthy of further investigation, and frontline musculoskeletal clinicians may find these additional questions useful to consider within the subjective history at an early stage in the patient journey. These items could inform the clinical reasoning process and raise the index of suspicion, helping to steer patients' on-going medical management.

The main reason for the development of the Christie Hospital checklist (2007) was that the clinicians had identified that patients were being referred late in the disease process. Late referral of these patients impacts very negatively on their quality of life. Levack et al (2002) highlight the significant problem of late diagnosis in MSCC, reporting that 82% (n = 205) of their patients were either unable to walk or could only do so with help at the time of diagnosis. They go on to state: *'The objective should be ... to diagnose MCC while patients are still walking'*.

A robust quantitative methodological framework has been developed for the production of clinical prediction

Table 2.1 A 2 × 2 table

		Disease	
		Positive	Negative
Test	Positive	True positive	False positive
	Negative	False negative	True negative

guides using four indices of test validity (Straus et al 2005):

- Sensitivity
- Specificity
- Positive predictive value
- Negative predictive value

These indices are used to construct a 2 × 2 table (Table 2.1), and this is very similar to the model of diagnostic alternatives that we have previously presented (Greenhalgh & Selfe 2006).

Sim & Wright (2000) state 'the sensitivity of a test is the extent to which it identifies those patients who do in fact have the disease (i.e. true positives), whereas the specificity of a test is the extent to which it fails to pick up those without the disease (i.e. true negatives). These can be calculated according to the following formulae (Farmer & Miller 1991):

Sensitivity
= true positives/(true positives + false negatives)

Specificity
= true negatives/(true positives + false positives)

Sensitivity and specificity both look at a population retrospectively over time whereas clinicians and patients are more interested in the need for a test to look to the future. The ideal test and the ideal Red Flag would perfectly discriminate between those with (true positive) and without disease (true negative). In reality, there can be overlap between those with and without disease, with false-positive and false-negative results commonly occurring (Schultz & Grimes 2006).

Unfortunately, although this is a well-established method, there appears to have been little work in applying this approach to Red Flags. Two papers have attempted to systematically investigate individual Red Flags: Harding et al (2005) investigated night pain and Buchanan et al (2006) investigated age under 20.

Harding et al (2005) conducted a prospective longitudinal study of 482 consecutive patients attending a back pain triage clinic to assess the importance of the symptom of night pain. A total of 213 patients reported night pain, with 90 reporting pain every night. Patients with night pain had 4.95 hours of continuous sleep (range 2–7) and were woken 2.5 times/night (range 0–6). No serious pathology was identified in any patient. Harding et al (2005) concluded:

> *'Although it is a significant and disruptive symptom for patients, these results challenge the specificity of the presence of night pain per se as a useful diagnostic indicator for serious spinal pathology in a back pain triage clinic.'*

In response to this paper, the CSP removed this item from the Red Flag list in its clinical guidelines on the physiotherapy management of persistent low back pain (CSP 2007).

Buchanan et al (2006) addressed the question:

'Is age less than 20 a useful Red Flag sign in low back pain?'

They reviewed the magnetic resonance imaging (MRI) database of a specialist orthopaedic hospital to establish the incidence of tumour and infection in 403 patients who presented to secondary care with low back pain; importantly it should be noted that the authors excluded patients who simultaneously presented any of the following co-morbidities:

- Neurological deficit
- Fever
- Acute deformity or scoliosis

The results demonstrated that 0.25% of young people with low back pain without simultaneous neurological deficit, fever, acute deformity or scoliosis had serious pathology. It is interesting to speculate whether this paper emphasizes that we need to look at combinations of co-morbidities, for example:

- Age <20 with neurological deficit
- Age <20 with fever
- Age <20 with acute deformity or scoliosis
- Or any of the other possible combinations of the above four variables.

However, from a practical point of view this would be a lengthy and costly study.

Both of the above papers provide important data, however, clinicians arriving at a diagnosis or prognosis rarely rely on a single sign, symptom or laboratory test. Waddell (2004) suggests that to arrive at an accurate and safe diagnosis, the key signs and symptoms need to be combined. The same is true for Red Flags. Klaber-Moffett et al (2006) state:

> *'clinicians should not uncritically accept any one red flag in isolation – the context is crucial.'*

Red Flags are essentially therefore clinical prediction guides; they are not diagnostic tests and they are not necessarily predictors of diagnosis or prognosis. In our view, the main role of Red Flags is that when combined, they to help to raise the clinician's index of suspicion.

We have attempted to highlight the clinical utility of this approach in our previous book by producing a hierarchical and weighted Red Flag list (Greenhalgh & Selfe 2006). Here, for ease of use, we present our updated list in the following section.

HIERARCHICAL LIST OF RED FLAGS

- Age >50 years + history of cancer + unexplained weight loss + failure to improve after 1 month of evidence-based conservative therapy

- Age <10 and >51

- Medical history (current or past) of:
  - Cancer
  - Tuberculosis
  - Human immunodeficiency virus (HIV) infection/ acquired immune deficiency syndrome (AIDS) or intravenous drug abuse
  - Osteoporosis
- Weight loss >10% body weight (3–6 months)
- Severe night pain precluding sleep
- Loss of sphincter tone and altered S4 sensation
- Bladder retention or bowel incontinence
- Positive extensor plantar response

🚩🚩

- Age 11–19
- Weight loss 5–10% body weight (3–6 months)
- Constant progressive pain
- Band-like pain
- Abdominal pain and changed bowel habits, but with no change of medication
- Inability to lie supine
- Bizarre neurological deficit
- Spasm
- Disturbed gait

🚩

- Loss of mobility, difficulty with stairs, falls, trips
- Legs misbehave, odd feelings in legs, legs feeling heavy
- Weight loss <5% body weight (3–6 months)
- Smoking
- Systemically unwell
- Trauma

- Bilateral pins and needles in hands and/or feet
- Previous failed treatment
- Thoracic pain
- Headache
- Physical appearance
- Marked partial articular restriction of movement

Using the example of Christine (Wardle et al 2007), who presented with what eventually proved to be a granulocytic sarcoma, we can compare the effect of applying our weighted Red Flag list with the unweighted list (CSAG 1994) (see Table 2.2).

The CSAG (1994) Red Flags:

Age of onset <20 or >55 years
Violent trauma, e.g. fall from a height, road traffic accident
Constant, progressive, non-mechanical pain
Thoracic pain
Past medical history of carcinoma
Systemic steroids
Drug abuse, HIV
Systemically unwell
Weight loss
Persistent, severe restriction of lumbar flexion
Widespread neurology
Structural deformity

Using Table 2.2 it is easy to see how the clinician's index of suspicion for Christine will be raised when using a weighted Red Flag list. This underlines the importance of looking at the patient from a holistic perspective and considering the context of each finding in

Table 2.2 Numbers of Red Flags present in the case of Christine

	CSAG (1994)	Greenhalgh & Selfe
Age 53		🚩🚩🚩
Constant non-mechanical pain	🚩	🚩🚩
Widespread neurology	🚩	🚩🚩
PMH carcinoma	🚩	🚩🚩🚩
Total Red Flags	3	10

PMH, past medical history.

light of other findings. This is further highlighted by Jalloh & Minhas (2007), who reported that in cases of cauda equina syndrome, there is a correlation between the time from presentation to surgery and the number of clinical features recorded at the initial assessment.

Crudely put, we could therefore say that the more Red Flags picked up at the initial consultation the better. However, there is clearly a tension here between being pragmatic in a clinical situation, where although 119 items in the subjective history and 44 items in the objective history have been identified as Red Flags (CSP 2007), it is highly unrealistic for clinicians to use all of these and still have time to actually manage their patients' conditions effectively.

References

Bigos S 1994 Acute low back pain in adults: clinical practice guideline. US Department of Health and Human Services, Rockville, MD, USA, AHCPR 95-0643

Buchanan E, Mukherjee K, Freeman R et al 2006 Is age less than 20 a useful 'Red Flag' sign in LBP. Nuffield Orthopaedic Centre, Oxford

Christie Hospital NHS Foundation Trust 2007 Spinal cord compression guidelines. Christie Hospital, Manchester

CSAG 1994 Report of a clinical standards advisory group on back pain. Her Majesty's Stationery Office, London

CSP 2007 Clinical guidelines for the effective physiotherapy management of persistent low back pain. CSP, London

Dawes M, Summerskill W, Glaziou P et al 2005 Sicily statement on evidence based practice. BMC Medical Education 5: 1

European Union 2004 European guidelines for prevention in low back pain. Online. Available: www.backpaineurope.org (accessed 28 January 2005)

Farmer R, Miller D 1991 Lecture notes on epidemiology and public health medicine, 3rd edn. Blackwell Scientific, Oxford

Greenhalgh S, Selfe J 2006 Red flags: a guide to identifying serious pathology of the spine. Churchill Livingstone, Elsevier, Edinburgh

Greenhalgh S, Selfe J 2008 Red flags for serious spinal pathology: a qualitative study of palliative care clinicians' opinion. Chartered Society of Physiotherapy, Annual Congress, Manchester

Guyatt G 1991 Evidence-based medicine. ACP Journal Club A–16: 114

Harding I J, Davies E, Buchanan E et al 2005 The symptom of night pain in a back pain triage clinic. Spine 30: 1985–1988

Henschke N, Maher C 2006 Red flags need more evaluation. Rheumatology 45: 920–921

Jalloh I, Minhas P 2007 Delays in the treatment of cauda equina syndrome due to its variable clinical features in patients presenting to the emergency department. Emergency Medicine Journal 24: 33–34

Jette D U, Ardleigh K, Chandler K et al 2006 Decision-making ability of physical therapists: physical therapy intervention or medical referral. Physical Therapy 86: 1619–1629

Klaber-Moffett J, McClean S, Roberts L 2006 Red flags need more evaluation: reply. Rheumatology 45: 921

Leerar P J, Boissonnault W G, Domholdt E et al 2007 Documentation of red flags by physical therapists for patients with low back pain. Journal of Manual and Manipulative Therapy 15: 42–49

Levack P, Graham J, Collie D et al 2002 Don't wait for a sensory level – listen to the symptoms: a prospective audit of the delays in diagnosis of malignant cord compression. Clinical Oncology 14: 472–480

New Zealand Ministry of Health 2004 New Zealand acute low back pain guidelines. Online. Available: www.nzgg.org.nz (accessed 4 April 2004)

National Institute for Health and Clinical Excellence 2001 Referral guidelines for low back pain. Online. Available: www.gp-training.net/rheum/backpain/index.htm (accessed 17 April 2008)

Overmeer T, Linton S J, Holmquist L et al 2005 Do evidence based guidelines have an impact in primary care? A cross-sectional study of Swedish physicians and physiotherapists. Spine 30: 146–151

Prodigy 2005 Low back pain. (Now Clinical Knowledge Summaries, http://cks.library.nhs.uk)

Roberts L, Fraser F, Murphy E A 2007 What is a Red Flag. World Confederation of Physical Therapy, Vancouver

Royal College of General Practitioners 2001 Clinical guidelines for the management of acute low back pain. Online. Available: www.rcgp.org.uk/clinspec/guidelines/backpain/index.asp (accessed 19 September 2007)

Sackett D L, Rosenberg W M C, Gray J A M et al 1996 Evidence based medicine: what it is and what it isn't. BMJ 312: 71–72

Schultz K F, Grimes D A 2006 The Lancet handbook of essential concepts in clinical research. Elsevier, Edinburgh

Sibbald B, Shen J, McBride A 2004 Changing the skill-mix of the health care workforce. Journal of Health Services Research and Policy 9: 28–38

Sim J, Wright C 2000 Research in health care. Nelson Thornes, Cheltenham

Straus E S, Richardson W S, Glaziou P et al 2005 Evidence-based medicine: how to practice and teach EBM, 3rd edn. Elsevier, Edinburgh

Waddell G 2004 The back pain revolution, 2nd edn. Churchill Livingstone, Edinburgh

Wardle F M, Maskell A P, Selfe J 2007 Christine: a case of granulocytic sarcoma of the upper trunk of the brachial plexus. Journal of Orthopaedic Medicine 29: 18–22

Wiesel S W, Weinstein J N, Herkowitz H et al 1996 The lumbar spine, International Society for the Study of the Lumbar Spine, 2nd edn. W B Saunders, Philadelphia

Chapter 3

Extra-pulmonary Spinal Tuberculosis

TWO CASES OF EXTRA-PULMONARY SPINAL TUBERCULOSIS

CASE 1: ALICE

The first time Alice was seen she was sitting fully clothed on a couch, waiting for the consultation. This was in June, eight months after her first onset of hip pain in the previous October. The room was well lit with magnolia-coloured walls, and the clinician's initial reaction was astonishment at how pale Alice looked compared with her surroundings. Despite her pallor Alice appeared relatively well, had managed to travel to the consultation by public transport, she could undress and dress comfortably, and she appeared like any other 18-year-old woman.

 What are you thinking now?

Alice had been referred by a general practitioner (GP) for pain radiating into the right thigh, which sometimes increased with coughing. The referral letter stated that she had a past medical history (PMH) of a road traffic accident (RTA) prior to the onset of symptoms (Figs 3.1, 3.2). Although Alice's stature aroused some comment and her haemoglobin was low at 9.2 g/dL (normal: approximately 14 g/dL), there were no other significant medical findings.

 What is your index of suspicion?

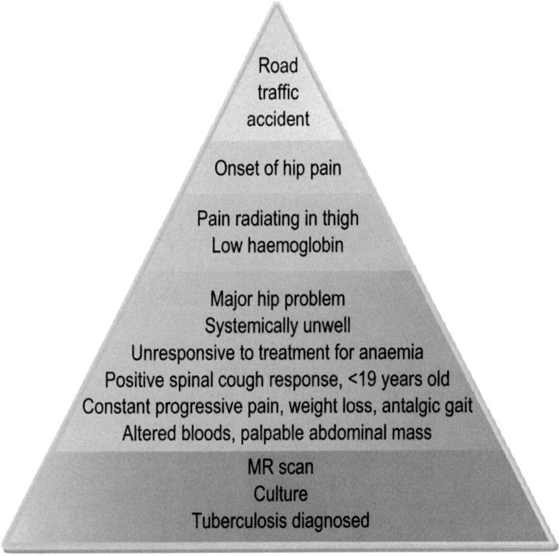

Road
traffic
accident

Onset of hip pain

Pain radiating in thigh
Low haemoglobin

Major hip problem
Systemically unwell
Unresponsive to treatment for anaemia
Positive spinal cough response, <19 years old
Constant progressive pain, weight loss, antalgic gait
Altered bloods, palpable abdominal mass

MR scan
Culture
Tuberculosis diagnosed

Fig. 3.1 Alice's journey from initial pain to diagnosis.

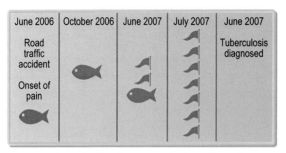

June 2006	October 2006	June 2007	July 2007	June 2007
Road traffic accident				Tuberculosis diagnosed
Onset of pain				

Fig. 3.2 Alice's timeline from onset of pain to diagnosis, including the number of Red Herrings and Red Flags.

At this first attendance at the triage service, it was noted that Alice had a significant problem with her gait, suggestive of an underlying right hip pathology, but the clinical examination was inconclusive. Alice had also by this time begun to experience some discomfort at night and walking distance had become limited to just five minutes before being forced to stop because of discomfort in the hip. Alice's mother raised some concern in relation to her possible weight loss but Alice herself described being well with minor loss of appetite. Despite a slight lumbar deviation to the right in standing, the lumbar spine and right hip examination were unremarkable, and it was the subjective history that led the clinician to take an X-ray of the right hip.

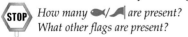 *How many* ⌁/⌁ *are present?*
What other flags are present?

At the second consultation one month later (July), when Alice attended for a review appointment and her

X-ray results, the presenting condition had changed considerably (Figs 3.1, 3.2). This time Alice had marked disturbance of sleep and malaise, with distinct loss of appetite. A marked cough response had developed with pain radiating on coughing from the lumbar and thoracic spine. The cough response was far more extreme in severity and extent of reference along the spinal column than the common cough response due to disc protrusion causing an increase in intra-thecal pressure. Alice's gait was grossly abnormal and yet her pelvic X-ray was unremarkable, apart from changes attributed to spasm in the right hip. Alice's GP had now prescribed iron tablets for anaemia, which Alice blamed for her constipation. Active lumbar spine left side flexion and extension were not possible; no neurological deficit was detected. Right hip examination was grossly abnormal with a marked fixed flexion contracture, however hip rotation remained normal.

Palpation of the abdomen revealed tenderness and possible mass in the right lower quadrant. Blood tests confirmed raised erythrocyte sedimentation rate (ESR) (84 mm/h; normal: approximately 5–15 mm/h) and C-reactive protein (CRP) (65 mg/L; normal: approximately <5 mg/L).

 What are your diagnostic alternatives?
What will you do next with this patient?

On the basis of these results, Alice was admitted for further investigation. Magnetic resonance imaging (MRI) of the spine identified signs of vertebral body osteomyelitis from T4 to T12 with signs of discitis at T10 and T11. There was a paraspinal mass under the anterior longitudinal ligament, which contrast enhancement identified as an abscess. There was an acute angular kyphosis at T10/11 with slight spinal cord impingement but no soft tissue mass within the vertebral canal.

What is challenging about this case?
What assumptions have you made about this case?
What is your level of plausibility and certainty?

The radiologist's impression was tuberculous discitis and tuberculous osteomyelitis, which was later confirmed by cell culture.

Alice was treated conservatively with combination chemotherapy, spinal bracing and drainage of the psoas abscess. Spinal bracing protected the stability of the spinal column and ensured the integrity of the spinal cord; it was continued for approximately 12 months.

CASE 2: BIBI

Bibi was a 23-year-old Asian woman who was born in England. She was very slight in build when she presented in June 2007 to an orthopaedic outpatient department. At the time of this initial consultation, her appetite was reduced, she was tired and very weak and distressed as a result of regular sleep disturbance due to buttock pain. Sustained positions and postures aggravated her pain, and this even included supine lying. On examination she was pale, gaunt and frail looking.

What are you thinking now?

One year previously (June 2006), Bibi had begun to have right buttock pain, radiating into the posterior thigh and extending to the posterior ankle. This changed over six months to include the sacro-iliac joint regions bilaterally. On referral from the physiotherapist to the orthopaedic clinic, a concern had been raised over Bibi's weight loss. Over a 12-month period she had accelerating weight loss, losing 3 kg in the first six months and 6 kg in the second six months (6 kg = 12% of her body weight). Her GP had initially referred Bibi to the physiotherapist in March 2007. The initial referral from the GP in March 2007 stated:

> *'She presents with no red flags.'*

At the initial GP consultation in February 2007, Bibi was described as having lumbo-sacral pain with some reference into the right leg and restricted forward flexion, but no neurological deficit. The letter went on to say that the GP had tried an evidence-based approach (Royal College of General Practitioners 2001), which had failed:

> *'She has been treated with standard Royal College of GP guidelines with analgesia and active rehabilitation, but continues to complain'*

 What is your index of suspicion?

At this GP consultation in February 2007, she was found to be anaemic (haemoglobin 7.9 g/dL; normal range: 11.5–16.5 g/dL) and was started on iron tablets (Figs 3.3, 3.4). Bibi's CRP was later found to be only slightly raised to 8.9 mg/L (normal: <5 mg/L) but her ESR was not tested. At the objective examination in the orthopaedic clinic in June 2007, flexion was the only grossly limited spinal movement, and straight leg raise on both left and right sides was limited (right 40 degrees, left 60 degrees) increasing back pain only and the right ankle jerk was absent. Bibi had not previously had low back pain or sciatica, and so this neurological

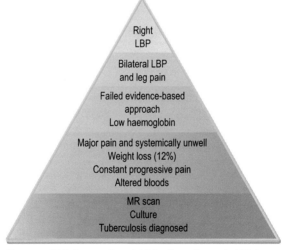

Fig. 3.3 Bibi's journey from initial pain to diagnosis. LBP, low back pain.

June 2006	March 2007	May 2007	June 2007	June 2007	July 2007
Onset of right buttock pain	GP reported no Red Flags	Physio-therapy	Extended Scope Physio-therapist	Oncologist	Tuberculosis diagnosed

Fig. 3.4 Bibi's timeline from onset of pain to diagnosis, including the number of Red Herrings and Red Flags.

deficit was likely to be clinically significant relative to the current episode. The clinician concluded that the S1 nerve root was being compromised but the number of Red Flags had raised the index of suspicion and therefore the conclusion of the greatest belief was that something serious could be the cause. As a consequence of this clinical reasoning, further blood investigations and an MRI scan were organized.

What are your diagnostic alternatives?
What is challenging about this case?

66

What assumptions have you made about this case?
What is your level of plausibility and certainty?

The MRI scan was carried out one week later and the report described a large tumour in the right sacral region. The tumour was described as growing through bone and soft tissue and through the foramen of the right S1 nerve root into the sacral canal. The tumour had crossed the midline and extended into the left piriformis muscle and adjacent fat. The images suggested a highly vascular and aggressive tumour.

 What will you do next with this patient?

Bibi was referred to a national bone tumour clinic regarded as a centre of excellence. At this centre it was concluded that this was not actually a malignant tumour, infection was suspected and extra-pulmonary tuberculosis suspected as the likely cause. A consultant chest physician later confirmed this in July 2007 by biopsy and histological examination at the local district general hospital (see Figs 3.3, 3.4) and prescribed a nine-month combination chemotherapy treatment package consisting of three drugs in line with the National Institute for Health and Clinical Excellence (NICE 2006) guidelines.

 What have you learnt from these cases?
Will you change your future practice?

TUBERCULOSIS

Tuberculosis is caused by *Mycobacterium tuberculosis* and is the oldest documented infectious disease – it was well known to Hippocrates. Sir Percival Pott gave a very good description of the disease in 1779; this description became a classic in the medical literature and spinal tuberculosis is still referred to as Pott's disease. In the past in Europe, pulmonary tuberculosis was called consumption, because it seemed to consume people from within. It was characterized by fever, haemoptysis and long, relentless wasting with sufferers appearing markedly pale. It was often associated with artistic creativity and romanticism (Dormanby 2001). The following extract from John Keats' poem *Ode to a Nightingale* captures the sense of this very well; Keats died of tuberculosis at the age of 26.

> *Fade far away, dissolve, and quite forget*
> *What thou among the leaves hast never known,*
> *The weariness, the fever, and the fret*
> *Here, where men sit and hear each other groan;*
> *Where palsy shakes a few, sad, last grey hairs,*
> *Where youth grows pale, and spectre-thin, and dies;*
> (Keats 1819)

Tuberculosis is a disease of poverty; the disease is more common in poor and deprived sections of society. It is the world's most prevalent and lethal infectious disease (Khoo et al 2003). According to the World Health Organization (WHO 2007), nearly a third (two billion people) of the world's population have tuberculosis, although many die with it rather than from it (WHO 2007). Tuberculosis is categorized as pulmonary or extra-pulmonary (or non-pulmonary), depending on the site of infection. However, all forms of the disease are initially contracted by the same air-borne route through the lungs. When people with active pulmonary tuberculosis cough, sneeze, speak, kiss or spit, they expel minute infectious droplets. A person with active but untreated pulmonary tuberculosis can infect 10–15 other people per year (WHO 2007).

Extra-pulmonary tuberculosis can affect any organ of the human body; the bacilli can be transported through the blood stream and lymph. The skeletal system is affected in 1–2% of cases if HIV negative; this rises to 60% if HIV positive (Khoo et al 2003). Of interest to musculoskeletal practitioners in the UK is that between 2004 and 2005 there was a larger percentage increase in the number of extra-pulmonary cases of tuberculosis reported (17%) compared with pulmonary cases (7%) (Health Protection Agency 2006).

The most common extra-pulmonary site for tuberculosis is the spine (Pott's disease), with the most common zone affected being T10 to L1. During a seven-year period in Blackburn in the northwest of England, there were 1072 cases of tuberculosis, 7% (n = 79) of which were extra-pulmonary bone and joint tuberculosis. The spine was the most commonly affected site with 44% of cases (3 cervical, 32 thoracolumbar and 1 sacro-iliac) (Sandher et al 2007). Griffith et al (2002) state that the majority of patients have two or more affected vertebrae by the time they are diagnosed. The anatomical area most affected is the anterior part of the vertebral body adjacent to the subchondral plate; the disease can then spread under the anterior longitudinal ligament. On plain X-rays, anterior destruction of the vertebral body with preservation of the disc space distinguishes tuberculosis from pyogenic infection (Miller 2004). Tuberculosis can cause destruction of several adjacent vertebral levels; in 10% of cases it can skip levels (Khoo et al 2003).

SUBJECTIVE EXAMINATION

Age/gender

- In the UK, most cases occur in young adults; 61% aged 15–44 (Alice, Bibi).
- In 2005, rates of disease in all age groups were higher among the non-UK-born population than in the UK-born population.
- The highest rates in the non-UK-born population were among those aged 25–29 years (179.6 per 100 000).
- Among the UK-born population, the highest rates occurred in the elderly (9.3 per 100 000 among those aged 80 years and over).
- In most of the world, tuberculosis affects more males than females. The UK infection rates are: males 16.6 per 100 000 and females 12.9 per 100 000.

(Health Protection Agency 2006)

In Africa, tuberculosis primarily affects adolescents and young adults. However, in developed countries where tuberculosis has gone from high to low incidence, it is mainly a disease of older people (WHO 2007).

Previous medical history

- HIV/AIDS
- Immune compromise
- Prolonged corticosteroid therapy and rheumatoid arthritis drugs
- Low body weight/undernourished/anorexia (Alice, Bibi)
- Alcoholism
- Diabetes mellitus
- Penetration of the body, e.g. needles, catheters or surgical procedures

(Bogduk & McGuirk 2002; Centers for Disease Control and Prevention 2007; Health Protection Agency 2006; WHO 2007)

Other less common conditions/factors to consider are:

- Silicosis
- Head and neck cancer
- Haematologic and reticuloendothelial disease, e.g. leukaemia and Hodgkin's disease
- End-stage kidney disease
- Intestinal bypass or gastrectomy
- Genetic disposition

(Centers for Disease Control and Prevention 2007; Ortega & Sanz-Gimeno 2004)

Tuberculosis is a leading killer among HIV-infected people with weakened immune systems; about 200 000 people living with HIV/AIDS die from tuberculosis every year. HIV/AIDS and tuberculosis are so closely connected that the term 'co-epidemic' or 'dual epidemic' is often used to describe their relationship. Because HIV affects the immune system, it increases the likelihood of people acquiring a new tuberculosis infection. HIV infection is also the most potent risk factor for converting latent tuberculosis into active tuberculosis, and infection with tuberculous bacteria accelerates the progress of AIDS infection in the patient. Each disease speeds up the progress of the other. Many people infected with HIV in developing countries develop tuberculosis as the first manifestation of AIDS (WHO 2007). It is interesting to note, however, in the recent study of Sandher et al (2007), no patients had HIV/AIDS or were immunosuppressed.

Drugs used in rheumatoid management work by blocking tumour necrosis factor alpha, increasing the risk of activating a latent tuberculosis infection, as this cytokine is very important in the immune response to tuberculosis.

Lifestyle/environment/geography

- Poor socio-economic conditions (Alice)
- Drug misuse
- Homelessness
- Migrants
- Healthcare workers
- In the UK in 2005, 43% of all cases reported were in London

(Centers for Disease Control and Prevention 2007; Health Protection Agency 2006; WHO 2007)

In response to changes made to the tuberculosis vaccination programme by the Department of Health in 2007, the health protection specialist in Bolton wrote to all parents and guardians of year 11 school pupils (15–16-year-olds) who were recorded as not having received bacille Calmette Guérin (BCG) immunization. This was to establish the need for screening and possible immunization. Screening was required if respondents answered yes to the following questions:

- Was your child born outside the UK with a rate of tuberculosis of at least 40 cases per 100 000 people (a list of countries was included)?
- Were your child's parents or grandparents born in a country with a rate of tuberculosis of at least 40 cases per 100 000 people?
- Is your child due to visit or live in a country with a rate of tuberculosis of at least 40 cases per 100 000 people for a period of one month or more?

In the context of this chapter, clinicians may find it useful to consider these additional questions during the subjective examination if extra-pulmonary tuberculosis is being considered as a diagnostic option. However, further work is needed to establish these as true risk factors for this particular condition (see Table 3.1).

Sandher et al (2007) report, in their series of 79 cases of extra-pulmonary tuberculosis, that eight patients were Caucasian, and 71 were non-white; only four of the non-white patients were born in the UK (Bibi).

Table 3.1 Estimated incidence of tuberculosis in 2005 (WHO 2007)

Country	Estimated incidence per 100 000 population
South Africa	600
Zambia	600
India	168
Thailand	142
Russian Federation	119
China	100
Brazil	60
Saudi Arabia	41
Portugal	33
Japan	28
Iran	23
UK	14
Finland	6.2
Australia	5.8
USA	4.5

History of current episode

- Gradual onset of back pain (Alice, Bibi)
- Local pain is often described as severe stabbing
- In cervical cases, pain may be referred to the occiput
- In thoracic cases, pain may manifest as intercostal neuralgia

- In the lumbar spine, pain may be referred to the hips and legs (Alice)
- Lethargy (Alice, Bibi)
- Fever
- Weight loss (Alice, Bibi)
- Evening rise in temperature
- Night sweats
- Night crying

(Duthie & Nelson 2000)

Bogduk & McGuirk (2002) reported that the cardinal indicator for an infection is fever; they went on to suggest that in cases where fever is present, clinicians should ask the question:

'Why should, or why could, this patient have an infection?'

In view of the very high endemic rates of tuberculosis, we recently asked some of our Zambian physiotherapy colleagues the following question:

'When a patient walks into the physiotherapy department for the first time complaining of back pain, what three questions would you ask in order to exclude/include extra-pulmonary TB [tuberculosis] as a diagnostic possibility?'

They replied (Mwango M, Mwila F, Nkandu E, personal communication 2008):

- How did the pain start?
  - Insidious onset

- Since starting with back pain, has your general health changed?
  - Malaise, fever, night sweats, loss of appetite
- What are the conditions (environment) like: at home, in the workplace or places you frequently visit?
  - Overcrowding, squalid, regular close contact with high-risk groups

OBJECTIVE EXAMINATION

- Local spinal pain
- May be kyphosis (Alice)
- Paravertebral swelling may be seen
- Antalgic posture of protective upright, stiff position (Alice). Sometimes referred to as 'boarding', this is the result of muscular rigidity and is one of the earliest clinical signs to appear
- Decreased range of motion (Alice, Bibi)
- If there is neural involvement there are likely to be neurological signs (may be widespread) (Bibi)
- Abscess sites should be examined: triangles of the neck, iliac fossae, groin, gluteal and ischial regions. Skin overlying the abscess may redden but not feel warm on palpation, leading to the term cold abscess
- A psoas abscess may present as a lump in the groin and resemble a hernia, or as a tender swelling below the inguinal ligament. A psoas abscess develops from a tubercular abscess in the lumbar vertebrae, which tracks inside the sheath of the psoas muscle (Alice)

(Duthie & Nelson 2000)

RED HERRINGS

- A psoas abscess can be confused with a hernia or enlarged inguinal lymph nodes.
- The spinal X-ray may be normal in early disease as 50% of the bone mass must be lost for changes to be visible on X-ray.
- Pallor associated with iron deficiency anaemia: this is usually caused by inadequate iron for haemoglobin synthesis. Tuberculosis causes a decreased release of iron from the bone marrow. Iron deficiency anaemia is usually responsive to traditional treatment such as improved diet and iron supplements (Kumar & Clark 2005).

DIFFERENTIAL DIAGNOSIS

Tuberculosis can be a difficult disease to diagnose (Alice, Bibi). This is sometimes due to the difficulty in culturing this slow-growing organism in the laboratory.

- Pyogenic infection
- Spinal tumours
- Infective discitis
- Acute bacterial osteomyelitis
- Septic arthritis

(Goel et al 2000; Sandher et al 2007; Vinas et al 2003)

If an infective process is suspected, the absence of BCG vaccination should raise the index of suspicion for tuberculosis (Sandher et al 2007).

GOLD STANDARD INVESTIGATIONS

- A needle biopsy from lymph nodes or pus aspirated from lymph nodes, pleura or any other surgical or radiological sample. If it shows tubercle bacilli, this is diagnostic but usually culture is required. Culture should include mycology (NICE 2006).
- Chest X-ray to check for co-existing respiratory tuberculosis (NICE 2006).
- In spinal tuberculosis, an early X-ray identifying vertebral body destruction anteriorly with preserved disc height distinguishes tuberculosis from pyogenic infections, which often show disc destruction.
- Elevated ESR. Laboratory investigations usually include a full blood count, ESR and CRP. The ESR is generally elevated in people with tuberculosis, but the leucocyte count may be normal (Perra & Winter 1996).
- Strongly positive Mantoux skin test.
- MRI may demonstrate the extent of spinal compression and can show changes at an early stage. Bone elements visible within the swelling, or abscesses, are strongly suggestive of Pott's disease rather than malignancy. Computed tomography (CT) and nuclear bone scans can also be used but MRI is best to assess risk to the spinal cord.

PATHOLOGY

Tuberculosis is not actually that easy to catch. It is usually estimated that eight hours of cumulative close contact is required. Most tuberculosis is post-primary and, as previously stated, the number of extra-pulmonary cases is increasing in the UK (Health Protection Agency 2006).

Progression from tuberculosis infection to tuber-culosis disease occurs when the tuberculous bacilli overcome the immune system defences and begin to multiply. In primary tuberculosis disease (1–5% of cases), this occurs soon after infection. However, in the majority of cases, a latent infection occurs that has no obvious symptoms. The dormant bacilli can produce tuberculosis in 2–23% of latent cases, often many years after infection (WHO 2007).

Gross pathological findings in tubercular spondylitis include granuloma and abscess formation. As abscesses develop, they coalesce, resulting in regions of necrosis containing the characteristic opaque, yellow 'cheesy' substance. These abscesses can follow tissue planes and at their margins they can form adhesions with visceral and vascular structures, which may become primary sources of symptoms including pain. In the neck, abscess formation may cause compression of the oesophagus and trachea. In the thoracic region, abscesses may form adhesions with the pleura or dia-phragm. Lumbar lesions may give rise to femoral abscess formation, and sacral abscesses can invade the perineum or the gluteal region through the greater sciatic foramen (Khoo et al 2003).

Timeline/prognosis

- Tuberculosis can remain dormant for 30–40 years
    - Once appropriate combination chemotherapy has been instigated, a cure is the most likely outcome
    - No tuberculosis deaths were recorded in the study of Sandher et al (2007)
    - Following appropriate treatment, 29% of the spinal patients had persistent back pain following treatment and four patients had a residual neurological deficit (Sandher et al 2007)
- Evidence-based treatment
    - Short course (six months) combination chemotherapy (NICE 2006). A combination of drugs helps overcome problems associated with drug resistance

SUMMARY

In a study conducted in Egypt, of 40 consecutive patients complaining of low back pain, who were attending a rheumatology service for their initial primary medical management, 12 were found to have extra-pulmonary tuberculosis as the cause of back pain. Clearly, this would not be the case in 2008, in an outpatient department in the northwest of England, but this highlights the need to understand the population trends within the area in which you work. Tuberculosis remains a significant cause of back pain in many parts of the world. In recent years, a lack of prevalence in the Western world due to successful medical management has led to a low index of suspicion generally in relation to tuberculosis (Abou-Raya & Abou-Raya 2006).

With increasing autonomy within physiotherapy practice, exposure to patients with non-pulmonary tuberculosis is likely to increase. Its insidious onset and prolonged prodromal phase can lead to the condition being missed with a number of clinicians being consulted before the ultimate diagnosis. Close multidisciplinary working between orthopaedic, thoracic medicine and pathology teams greatly facilitates diagnosis (Sandher et al 2007). Bibi's case in particular highlights the challenge of diagnosing extra-pulmonary tuberculosis, as this final diagnosis was reached following consulting at least five different competent clinicians in different medical specialties. It is important to note that all the clinicians involved with Bibi acted within current best practice guidelines and in a timely fashion, yet it took approximately 13 months to reach a definitive diagnosis. Interestingly, Khoo et al (2003) reported that in industrialized countries the diagnosis of tuberculosis can take up to two years after the onset of symptoms. Bibi illustrates how an elongated prodromal phase can be misleading but how the post-prodromal timeline of the disease often displays a rapid progression.

The important similarities between the two case histories presented here are the insidious onset of pain, low initial body weight combined with weight loss for no

apparent reason and anaemia – symptoms strongly suggestive of systemic pathology. It is also important to
highlight Alice's very poor socio-economic status and
environmental conditions as potential contributing
factors to her condition.

References

Abou-Raya S, Abou-Raya A 2006 Spinal tuberculosis
overlooked? Journal of Internal Medicine 260: 160–163
Bogduk N, McGuirk B 2002 Medical management of acute and
chronic low back pain: an evidence based approach. Elsevier,
Amsterdam
Centers for Disease Control and Prevention 2007 Tuberculosis
fact sheet. Online. Available: www.cdc.gov/tb (accessed 25
September 2007)
Dormanby T 2001 The white death: a history of tuberculosis.
The Hambledon Press, London
Duthie R B, Nelson C L 2000 Infections of the musculoskeletal
system. In: Duthie R B, Bentley G (eds) Mercer's orthopaedic
surgery, 9th edn. Hodder Arnold, London
Goel V, Young J B, Patterson C J 2000 Infective discitis as an
uncommon but important cause of back pain in older
people. Age and Ageing 29: 454–456
Griffith J F, Kumta S M, Leung P C et al 2002 Imaging of
musculoskeletal tuberculosis: a new look at an old
disease. Clinical Orthopaedics and Related Research 398:
32–39
Health Protection Agency 2006 Focus on tuberculosis: annual
surveillance report – England, Wales and Northern Ireland.
Health Protection Agency, London
Keats J 1819 Ode to a Nightingale. Online. Available:
www.poetry-online.org/keats_ode_to_a_nightingale.htm
(accessed 19 September 2007)
Khoo L T, Mikawa K, Fessler R G 2003 A surgical revisitation of
Pott distemper of the spine. Spine Journal 3: 130–145

Kumar P, Clark M 2005 Clinical medicine, 6th edn. W B
    Saunders, Edinburgh
Miller M D 2004 Review of orthopaedics, 4th edn. W B
    Saunders, Edinburgh
Mwango M, Mwila F, Nkandu E 2008 Subjective examination of
    LBP in Zambia. Personal communication
National Institute for Health and Clinical Excellence 2006
    Tuberculosis. Clinical diagnosis and management of
    tuberculosis, and measures for its prevention and control.
    NICE, London
Ortega J A, Sanz-Gimeno A 2004 Siblings in death: concordance
    in siblings' cause of death in Aranjez (1871–1970). Colloque,
    freres-soeurs-jumeaux. Passe et present des fratries, Lyon
Perra J H, Winter R B 1996 Spinal infection: when to suspect it
    and how to manage it. Journal of Musculoskeletal Medicine
    13: 15–23
Royal College of General Practitioners 2001 Clinical guidelines
    for the management of acute low back pain. Online.
    Available: www.rcgp.org.uk/clinspec/guidelines/backpain/
    index.asp (accessed 19 September 2007)
Sandher D S, Al-Jibury M, Paton R W et al 2007 Bone and joint
    tuberculosis: cases in Blackburn between 1988 and 2005.
    Journal of Bone and Joint Surgery (Br) 89: 1379–1381
Vinas C F, Rhodes R, Giger A 2003 Spinal infections. Online.
    Available: www.emedecine.com/orthoped (accessed 22 April
    2004)
WHO 2007 Tuberculosis infection and transmission. Online.
    Available: www.who.int/mediacentre/factsheets/fs104/en/
    (accessed 19 September 2007)

Chapter 4

Cauda Equina Syndrome

TWO CASES OF CAUDA EQUINA SYNDROME

CASE 1: CLARE

Clare was a 35-year-old woman, urgently referred in January 2006. She began with low back pain approximately two years before, in 2004. The onset of symptoms was gradual, but at that time (2004) she had no leg pain and her symptoms resolved spontaneously. The current episode of pain had been the most severe to date. It began in October 2005, the symptoms gradually deteriorated over the subsequent three months, but had deteriorated more rapidly over the last month. Pain control had been difficult as Clare suffered from irritable bowel syndrome and biliary gastritis, which militated against adequate medication for pain control.

Initially the symptoms were in the lumbar spine. They then spread to Clare's right leg, and over the previous month had also spread to her left leg as well. At a party in December 2005, the symptoms deteriorated further. The bilateral leg pain became much more severe, particularly in the calves. Clare had no pins and needles or numbness and the reference of pain was symmetrical, but more severe on the right. A cough and sneeze increased leg pain and the symptoms were aggravated by lying supine and eased by crook lying with the right hip flexed, close to tissue approximation to her chest. Over the previous week her legs had felt very heavy and weak. Clare reported episodes of bladder and bowel dysfunction, particularly over the past month. She had one episode of faecal incontinence, but attributed this to her irritable bowel syndrome, which she had been diagnosed with some years earlier, and so for which she did not seek help. Clare also reported episodes of intermittent urinary retention, with one episode lasting a full day. Clare felt that on occasions when she attempted to micturate, she was unable to push and could not completely empty her bladder.

 What are you thinking now?

On examination, Clare was obviously struggling and in marked pain. She was standing in flexion with left-sided spinal deviation and the right knee flexed. Clare was very slight in build, which enabled the clinician to see the L5 spinous process, which unusually appeared to be slightly prominent. In standing, the pain extended down to both calves, the right being worse than the left. She had no spinal extension, very limited spinal flexion and leg pain was increased by right side flexion. She had no straight leg raise on the right. In supine lying, passive extension of the right knee was not possible due to pain and neural tension signs. Straight leg raise on the left was to 20 degrees, increasing left leg pain. Femoral nerve stretch was not tested, as Clare was very uncomfortable and unable to lie prone. She had some weakness of right dorsi-flexion and eversion with slight blunting of the right ankle jerk. The spinous process of L5 did appear to be more prominent even in side lying. Clare did have the ability to slightly contract the gluteal muscles; further examination revealed that she had poor anal sphincter tone.

What is your index of suspicion?
How many ◑/◢ are present?
What are your diagnostic alternatives?
What is your level of plausibility and certainty?

Claire had previously had investigations for a urinary tract infection, but to her knowledge these were negative. The clinician's impression was that Clare had a large central prolapsed intervertebral disc, possibly the L4/5 disc, compromising the L5 roots bilaterally and compromising the cauda equina. The patient underwent magnetic resonance imaging (MRI) as an emergency according to the cauda equina protocol (Fig. 4.1).

The MRI confirmed the presence of a large right para-central disc prolapse at L4/5 with compression of both L5 nerve roots and crowding but not compression of the cauda equina.

What will you do next with this patient?

Consequently, Claire was admitted as an emergency and underwent spinal surgery. We are happy to report

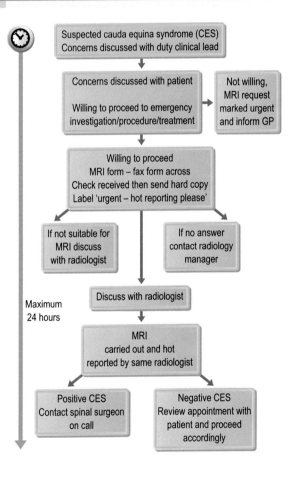

Suspected cauda equina syndrome (CES)
Concerns discussed with duty clinical lead

Concerns discussed with patient

Willing to proceed to emergency
investigation/procedure/treatment

Not willing,
MRI request
marked urgent
and inform GP

Willing to proceed
MRI form – fax form across
Check received then send hard copy
Label 'urgent – hot reporting please'

If not suitable for
MRI discuss
with radiologist

If no answer
contact radiology
manager

Discuss with radiologist

MRI
carried out and hot
reported by same radiologist

Positive CES
Contact spinal surgeon
on call

Negative CES
Review appointment with
patient and proceed
accordingly

Maximum
24 hours

that further communication with the patient revealed that she made a full recovery.

 What is challenging about this case?
What assumptions did you make about this case?

CASE 2: DEBBIE

Debbie was a 40-year-old woman seen on an urgent basis with an acute and progressing nerve root entrapment. Debbie had a five-year history of intermittent low back pain with right-sided sciatica. The symptoms usually resolved spontaneously. However, at Christmas in 2005 she experienced an episode of low back pain and right sciatica with pins and needles in the right calf. This progressed to bilateral leg pain, which then changed to the left leg with posterior heel pain and paraesthesia. Worryingly, symptoms continued to progress to saddle numbness and hesitancy of bladder function but no episodes of complete urinary retention. Over the previous week Debbie described a sudden improvement in pain, but the saddle numbness and bladder hesitancy remained marked.

 What are you thinking now?

Examination revealed a good range of spinal movement with no restriction of neural mobility, but right ankle jerk was absent. Sensation was reduced in the

Fig. 4.1 Clinical Assessment, Treatment and Support (CATS) cauda equina protocol (Winters et al 2006). (Redrawn with permission from Bolton PCT.)

lateral aspect of the left calf, but more importantly sensation was reduced in the left saddle region and left buttock. The anal reflex appeared to be absent, but Debbie did have some active contraction and sphincter tone on per rectum (PR) examination.

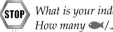 *What is your index of suspicion?*
How many */* *are present?*

The clinician suspected that the cauda equina was at risk of being compromised, probably by an L5/S1 disc.

 What are your diagnostic alternatives?
What is your level of plausibility and certainty?
What will you do next with this patient?

The clinician acted according to the cauda equina protocol (see Fig. 4.1) and requested an urgent MRI scan. This confirmed a large central to right L5/S1 disc compromising the cauda equina. Debbie was admitted as an emergency and spinal surgery was carried out.

 What is challenging about this case?
What assumptions did you make about this case?

CAUDA EQUINA SYNDROME

Within the musculoskeletal field, urinary retention is a well-known symptom identified in the subjective history that would alert the clinician to cauda equina syndrome (CES), the most common cause being discal in origin. However, a focus group held with experienced palliative care clinicians from a hospice in the northwest of England also highlighted the importance of bowel dysfunction. These clinicians suggested that faecal incontinence could be an initial presenting symptom of serious pathology associated with malignant spinal cord compression (MSCC) (Greenhalgh & Selfe 2008). The importance of this point is supported by Markham (2004), who argued that any combination of bladder and bowel dysfunction should alert the clinician to CES. There are two main causes of CES:

- Prolapsed intervertebral disc
- Malignant spinal cord compression

As CES is defined as a medical emergency, it is mandatory that clinicians should routinely ask about bladder and bowel functions during the subjective examination (Clinical Standards Advisory Group (CSAG) 1994; New Zealand Ministry of Health 2004; Royal College of General Practitioners 2001). In the UK patients tend to fall into two groups: those who are extremely reticent in talking about these kinds of symptoms and those who seem to like nothing better than giving you a detailed account of their toilet habits and functions. Not only is there a potential for the patient to be embarrassed discussing these presenting symptoms, this sensitive, yet crucial questioning can also be challenging for the clinician.

PROLAPSED INTERVERTEBRAL DISC

The term cauda equina (horse's tail) refers to the sheaf of nerve roots which descend within the spinal canal distal to the conus medullaris, the termination of the spinal cord, which is approximately at the L1–L2 level (Williams et al 2003). Compression of these roots can cause a variety of motor and sensory neural problems of the lower limbs, pelvic viscera and pelvic floor function (Wiesel et al 1996). However, the most significant problem is considered to be the compromise of the cauda equina (typically the fourth sacral root), which leads to interruption in bladder and bowel function and is potentially irreversible (Brier 1999; Cyriax 1982). Once a patient presents with established CES, surgical procedures are less likely to reverse the impaired bladder/bowel and sexual function due to the timeline that has precipitated these symptoms (Caputo & Cusimano 2002).

In cases where bladder and bowel symptoms are reported, it is important to establish the chronology between these and the onset of low back pain (Sapsford & Kelly 2004). It is also important to establish the chronology of certain medications administered and the onset of bladder dysfunction; see Red Herrings later in this chapter (BMJ 2007). Careful questioning can help to prevent unnecessary alarm and inappropriate investigations where other non-emergency causes of altered bladder and bowel functions have occurred prior to the onset of low back pain, for example post partum.

Although a clinically important condition, CES is quite rare, with the prevalence among all back patients being estimated at 0.0004 (Jarvik & Deyo 2002), and an annual incidence estimated at 1 in 33000–100000 (Caputo & Cusimano 2002). In the UK it has been estimated that only one CES case will present annually for every 50 000 patients seen in primary care settings (Office of National Statistics 1995). In 2005 the Clinical Assessment, Treatment and Support (CATS) service in Bolton (Greater Manchester, UK) saw six such cases from a population of 275 000. It is a complication of approximately 2% of lumbar disc herniation cases (Winters et al 2006).

Although CES is uncommon, it is associated with a high level of litigation. Markham (2004) highlighted 96 cases of CES notified to the Medical Defence Union in the UK; 65% of these progressed to claims by the patients and nearly half of these resulted in compensation payments. Unlike many of the other conditions we discuss in this book, acute CES associated with intervertebral disc prolapse does not generally demonstrate an extended prodromal period where low-grade symptoms can smoulder for months or even years. However, as Jalloh & Minhas (2007) argue, and in common with many other serious pathology, the fewer signs and symptoms that the patient presents with, the more likely is CES to be missed.

MALIGNANT SPINAL CORD COMPRESSION

Malignant spinal cord compression can lead to a variety of problems including:

- Urinary retention
- Constipation
- Urinary and faecal incontinence
- Post-voiding large residual volume

This bladder and bowel dysfunction can be divided into two categories (Christie Hospital NHS Foundation Trust 2007):

- Reflex bladder
- Flaccid bladder

A reflex bladder is also known as a spastic bladder or an automatic bladder and occurs as a result of spinal cord compression above T12. When the bladder is full, it may empty automatically. As the nerves above the sacral region of the spinal cord no longer communicate with the brain, the patient will have no sensation of a full bladder. A similar problem can occur with the bowel if the spinal cord is compressed above T12 leading to a spastic bowel. The bowel can contract and empty when stimulated; importantly, anal sphincter tone is retained.

When cord compression occurs below the level of T12 and affects the sacral region of the spinal cord, all reflexes are affected and the bladder will lose muscle tone, resulting in a flaccid bladder. The resulting incontinence is an overflow incontinence; as the bladder overfills, patients have no sensory awareness of a full bladder. Similarly a flaccid bowel may develop where there is faecal retention and overflow of faecal material with flaccid anal sphincter tone.

SUBJECTIVE EXAMINATION

According to Cyriax (1982) 'It is a full history rather than the examination which inspires caution' in cases of

CES. The following items have been suggested by the Christie Hospital (2007) as appropriate prompts for questioning patients with suspected CES in primary care settings:

- When urine was last voided
- Episodes of incontinence
- Symptoms of urgency, frequency or retention
- Abdominal pain and/or distention
- Fluid intake
- Frequency and consistency of stools
- Nausea/vomiting
- Abdominal pain or distension
- Dietary and drug history

Levack et al (2002) in their study of MSCC, reported that 56% (n = 139) of patients reported having at least one problem with passing urine.

Age/gender

- More prevalent among men in the fourth and fifth decade of life
- <50 years, consider discal origin (Clare, Debbie)
- >50 years, consider serious pathology
- Not race specific

(MD Consult 2007; Small et al 2005)

Previous medical history

Previous carcinoma (Greenhalgh & Selfe 2008; Levack et al 2002; Waddell 2004).

Lifestyle/environment/geography

Human immunodeficiency virus (HIV) infection (Waddell 2004).

History of current episode (see Table 4.1)

- Back pain with nerve root distribution of pain (one or more nerve roots involved) (Clare)
- Sciatica (a report of bilateral sciatica is often considered particularly important in cases of CES) (Clare, Debbie)
- Saddle paraesthesia and/or anaesthesia around the anus, perineum or genitals (Debbie)
- Insensitivity to urine passing down the urethra during micturition
- Faecal incontinence (Clare)
- Bladder dysfunction, e.g. urinary retention with or without overflow incontinence, difficulty voiding (Clare, Debbie)

Table 4.1 Sensitivity of symptoms of cauda equina sydrome (Deyo et al 1992)

	Sensitivity
Urinary retention	0.90
Unilateral or bilateral sciatica	>0.80
Sensory/motor deficit and reduced SLR	>0.80
Saddle anaesthesia	0.75

SLR, straight leg raising.

- Sexual dysfunction, e.g. erectile dysfunction, and, in females, dyspareunia (pain during intercourse)
- Weak/heavy legs (Clare)
- Gait disturbance
- Systemically unwell

(Bartley 2001; Brier 1999; Duthie 1996; Greenhalgh & Selfe 2008; Royal College of General Practitioners 2001; Souhami & Tobias 1995; Waddell 2004)

OBJECTIVE EXAMINATION

- Decreased anal sphincter tone (60–80% cases) (Clare, Debbie)
- Sacral sensory loss (85% cases (n = 27))

(Jalloh & Minhas 2007)

We would like to emphasize that during the clinical examination of anal tone and peri-anal sensations, sufficient training and competency of the clinician is essential.

RED HERRINGS

- Medication, e.g. amitriptyline, tramadol and other morphine salts. Side effects include constipation and difficulty with micturition
- Stress incontinence
- Pain-induced hesitancy, especially in men
- Urinary tract infection (Clare)

(BMJ Publishing Group 2007; Levack et al 2002)

DIFFERENTIAL DIAGNOSIS

- Disc (Clare, Debbie)
- Infection
- Tumour – malignant or benign usually extending from a vertebral body
- Upper motor neurone lesion
- Trauma

(Brier 1999; Souhami & Tobias 1995)

GOLD STANDARD INVESTIGATIONS

MRI is the recommended diagnostic test for CES (Waddell 2004). See Figure 4.1 for example of a clinical management protocol.

PATHOLOGY

The anatomical features of the cauda equina predispose it to symptoms of compression. The nerve roots in this area are covered in a sparse layer of connective tissue as opposed to the thick epineurium found in peripheral nerves, offering little protection against tensile forces. This along with a lack of regionalized segmental blood supply compounds the vulnerability of this anatomical region (Caputo & Cusimano 2002).

The most common cause of CES is a central disc prolapse which occupies all or most of the spinal canal compressing all lumbar and sacral nerves at that level and lower levels of the spinal column (Marks 2006).

Compression of these nerves leads to potential loss of sphincter tone, incomplete emptying of the bladder, and compromise of the stretch receptors and/or difficulty initiating micturition or defecation (Brown 1998).

Timeline/prognosis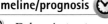

⊙ Delays in treatment of CES are most often because of delay in making the diagnosis. Predictably, this is more likely when fewer features of CES are established at the time of presentation (Jalloh & Minhas 2007).

EVIDENCE-BASED TREATMENT

Emergency referral for surgical opinion for consideration of necessity for urgent decompression (Acre et al 2001). It has been established that early diagnosis and operative management within 48 hours of sphincter disturbance lead to better outcome than a non-surgical management (Jalloh & Minhas 2007).

If CES goes undetected in the initial phase, the appropriate management gets delayed leading to an increase in morbidity (Jalloh & Minhas 2007).

SUMMARY

A number of interesting comparisons can be made between Clare and Debbie. Although both cases were caused by lumbar disc prolapse, they were at different levels, which probably accounts for the variation in symptoms. Both patients reported intermittent low back pain over at least two years, but neither had experienced these types of symptoms previously. Clinicians should be particularly alert to any alterations in the 'usual' pattern of pain or dysfunction in cases like these, where previous episodes of low back pain have occurred. One of the main clinical features to note in these two cases is the contrast in pain levels at the time of consultation: Clare was in severe pain but Debbie's low back pain had completely resolved. However, both patients still had numerous, well-developed Red Flags for CES; in particular, both patients complained of bladder dysfunction and both had decreased anal sphincter tone. Additionally, it is interesting to note the Red Herrings present in Clare's case, where she misattributed her faecal incontinence to her irritable bowel syndrome and she was tested for a urinary tract infection.

Despite the diverse nature of these two cases, the crucial timing of an emergency surgical opinion remains the same. In the case of the Bolton CATS cauda equina protocol (Fig. 4.1), the timing is a maximum of 24 hours from the first clinical suspicion that cauda equina symptoms may be present. If you are suspicious that the patient may have CES, it may be appropriate to initiate further investigation and seek an emergency surgical opinion. It is essential to establish your own local pathway before these cases present.

References

Acre D, Sass P, Abul-Khoudoud H 2001 Recognising spinal cord emergencies. American Family Physician 64: 631–638

Bartley R 2001 Nerve root compression and cauda equina syndrome. In: Bartley R, Coffey P (eds) Management of low back pain in primary care. Butterworth Heinemann, Oxford, pp 63–67

BMJ Publishing Group 2007 BNF, September edn. BMJ Publishing Group & RPS Publishing, London

Brier S R 1999 Primary care orthopaedics. Mosby, St Louis

Brown K L 1998 Cauda equina syndrome: implications for the orthopaedic nurse in a clinical setting. Orthopaedic Nursing 17: 31–35

Caputo L A, Cusimano M D 2002 Atypical presentation of cauda equina syndrome. Journal of the Canadian Chiropractic Association 46: 31–38

Christie Hospital NHS Foundation Trust 2007 Spinal cord compression guidelines. Christie Hospital, Manchester

Clinical Standards Advisory Group 1994 Report of a clinical standards advisory group on back pain. Her Majesty's Stationery Office, London

Cyriax J 1982 Textbook of orthopaedic medicine, 8th edn. Baillière Tindall, Eastbourne

Deyo R A, Rainville J, Kent D L 1992 What can the history and physical examination tell us about low back pain? Journal of the American Medical Association 268: 760–765

Duthie R B 1996 Affections of the spine. In: Duthie R B (ed) Mercer's orthopaedic surgery, 9th edn. Arnold, London, pp 915–1014

Greenhalgh S, Selfe J 2008 Red flags for serious spinal pathology: a qualitative study of palliative care clinicians' opinion. Chartered Society of Physiotherapy, Annual Congress, Manchester

Jalloh I, Minhas P 2007 Delays in the treatment of cauda equina syndrome due to its variable clinical features in patients presenting to the emergency department. Emergency Medicine Journal 24: 33–34

Jarvik J G, Deyo R A 2002 Diagnostic evaluation of low back pain with emphasis on imaging. Annals of Internal Medicine 137: 586–597

Levack P, Graham J, Collie D et al 2002 Don't wait for a sensory level – listen to the symptoms: a prospective audit of the delays in diagnosis of malignant cord compression. Clinical Oncology 14: 472–480

Markham D E 2004 Cauda equina syndrome: diagnosis, delay and litigation risk. Journal of Orthopaedic Medicine 26: 102–105

Marks S 2006 The cauda equina syndrome. Clinical Risk 12: 25–28

MD Consult 2007 Cauda equina syndrome. Online. Available: www.mdconsult.com (accessed 13 December 2007)

New Zealand Ministry of Health 2004 New Zealand acute low back pain guidelines. Online. Available: www.nzgg.org.nz (accessed 4 April 2003)

Office of National Statistics 1995 Morbidity statistics from general practice. Fourth national study 1991–1992. Her Majesty's Stationery Office, London

Royal College of General Practitioners 2001 Clinical guidelines for the management of acute low back pain. Online. Available: www.rcgp.org.uk/clinspec/guidelines/backpain/index.asp (accessed 19 September 2007)

Sapsford S, Kelly S 2004 Pelvic floor dysfunction in low back and sacroiliac dysfunction. In: Boyling J D, Hull G A (eds) Grieve's modern manual therapy, 3rd edn. Elsevier, Edinburgh

Small S A, Perron A, Brady W J 2005 Orthopaedic pitfalls: cauda equina syndrome. American Journal of Emergency Medicine 23: 159–163

Souhami R, Tobias J 1995 Cancer and its management, 2nd edn. Blackwell, Oxford

Waddell G 2004 The back pain revolution, 2nd edn. Churchill Livingstone, Edinburgh

Wiesel S W, Weinstein J N, Herkowitz H et al 1996 The lumbar spine, 2nd edn. W B Saunders, Philadelphia

Williams P L, Bannister L H, Berry M M et al 2003 Gray's anatomy, 38th edn. Churchill Livingstone, New York

Winters M E, Klutetz P, Zilberstein J 2006 Back pain emergencies. Medical Clinics of North America 90: 505–523

Chapter 5

Cancer

This chapter is presented in a slightly different format to the others as it is split into two sections. The first section presents a case history of a patient with spinal metastases and then specifically discusses breast cancer followed by malignant spinal cord compression. The second section presents two case histories of patients with multiple myeloma and then goes on to discuss general issues associated with cancer.

METASTATIC DISEASE (SECONDARY DISEASE)

CASE 1: EDITH

Edith was a 71-year-old woman who had a previous history of breast cancer. She presented to an orthopaedic triage service in November 2001. She had been referred by her general practitioner (GP). Edith had started to have thoracic pain in the previous August, and the onset was gradual. The pain began in the upper right thoracic region extending around the lateral aspect of the rib cage to the anterior chest and was progressing down the arm in a T1 distribution. Painkillers were not helping and Edith attributed her general feeling of being unwell to these. In addition, Edith was using an anti-inflammatory gel, but this was also ineffective; in fact Edith reported that she could not stand the pressure of the gel being rubbed in. Pain was constant and aggravated by any activity, but it eased with rest, but the pain never went away completely. A cough and sneeze were negative. First thing in the morning, the pain was tolerable for a short time but then increased. Edith was able to sleep but only when lying on the left side. She could not tolerate any pressure on the thoracic spine when lying supine or on the right side. Bladder and bowel function remained normal, although she had developed constipation which she attributed to her drugs. She described herself as feeling poorly. Edith was only slight in stature yet she reported a significant amount of weight loss which her husband confirmed as being approximately 9 kg (1.5 stone) over the past six weeks.

 What are you thinking now?

Objective examination was carried out in standing and sitting as lying was so uncomfortable. Interestingly, the range of motion of both thoracic and lumbar spines was normal for her age. Palpation using postero-anterior pressure over the spinous processes in sitting did not aggravate the pain, however light palpation over the right ribs anteriorly was exquisitely painful. No neurological deficit was detected. A scoliosis convex to the left was observed in the lumbar spine with a thoracic curve convex to the right. Both Edith and her husband were very distressed by the rapid deterioration in her condition and were desperate for help.

 What is your index of suspicion?
How many ☞/☞ are present?

The clinician was very concerned about Edith in view of her age, weight loss, thoracic pain, previous history of mastectomy, progressive pain and raised erythrocyte sedimentation rate (ESR) of 41 mm/h (normal reported range = 5–15 mm/h).

 What are your diagnostic alternatives?
What will you do next with this patient?

The orthopaedic consultant on call was contacted and the clinical picture including the concerning features described. Edith was sent home following a repeat blood test for ESR and a bone scan was arranged. The blood test result showed that ESR had risen slightly to 45 mm/h and the bone scan report stated that there were

'focal areas of isotope uptake, particularly around the anterior aspects of the 3rd, 4th, 5th and 6th ribs.'

The bone scan report also stated that

'these findings were consistent with previous trauma or fractures.'

In addition there was an increased uptake of isotope at T5. In the report there was some debate as to whether this was due to thoracic scoliosis and multiple degenerative changes. Edith was immediately admitted onto an orthopaedic ward for further investigations and pain control. The subjective history had confirmed that no previous trauma to the ribs had ever occurred, either recently or in the past.

 What is your index of suspicion?

Unfortunately at this admission, it was confirmed that the increased uptake at T5 was related to metastatic activity.

Edith's case clearly illustrates how Red Flags can raise the clinician's index of suspicion and demonstrates that the larger the combination of Red Flags, the more focused is the conclusion of greatest belief. On assimilating the information in this case history, the reader undoubtedly had a high index of suspicion. It is interesting, therefore, to recognize that the serious cause for Edith's pain was not identified by two competent clinicians who saw Edith very early in her disease process when she presented with few Red Flags. In fact, in the early stages she had only two Red Flags:

- Age
- Previous history of breast cancer

At that time, her pain was intermittent, not constant or progressive, she had no weight loss, she generally felt well and in good health and her ESR was within normal limits. Imagine the case history now with this different combination of Red Flags.

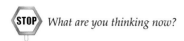 *What are you thinking now?*

In this earlier version of Edith's case history, the reader's index of suspicion is much lower.

Summary

Although the course of Edith's illness probably would not have been changed, with a speedier diagnosis Edith's symptom management could have been improved (National Institute for Health and Clinical Excellence (NICE) 2008).

CANCER

More than 10 million people are diagnosed with cancer every year. It is estimated that there will be 15 million new cases every year by 2020. Currently cancer causes six million deaths per year or 12% of deaths worldwide; the chance of cure, however, increases substantially if cancer is detected early (World Health Organization (WHO) 2004).

The WHO International Agency for Research on Cancer (WHO 2004) estimates that 10% of all cancer deaths in non-smokers are related to obesity. The relationship between increased cancer risk is approximately linear with increasing body mass index and decreasing physical activity. Obesity and inactivity account for a quarter to a third of the cancers of the breast, colon, endometrium, kidney and oesophagus. The most common cancers worldwide are (WHO 2004):

- Lung – men
- Stomach – men
- Breast – women
- Cervical – women

Osteoblastomas are rare, benign tumours which can occur in the vertebrae. These lesions occur more frequently in men than in women, by a ratio of 1.5–4:1. Osteoblastomas are most painful at night, with the pain being dramatically relieved by aspirin. Treatment is curettage, with bone grafting if necessary, and treatment usually cures the condition (Abbott et al 2003).

Metastatic spinal disease

The cancers most commonly seeding metastases to the spine are:

- Breast
- Prostate
- Lung

The five-year survival rates for prostate and breast cancer in Australia are now greater than 80% (Australian Department of Health and Ageing 2004). The five-year survival rate for prostate cancer is greater than 50% and breast cancer greater than 75% in 16 European cancer registries (European Commission 2004).

BREAST CANCER

As the most common cancer to seed metastases to the spine is breast cancer, we thought it would be helpful to specifically review breast cancer here. One of the clinical patterns that is important to consider here is when breast cancer has previously been undiagnosed and the patient seeks medical or therapeutic intervention for the musculoskeletal effects of metastases; we have previously published a case history (of Margaret) who presented exactly in this way (Greenhalgh & Selfe 2004).

Subjective examination

- Family history in first-degree relative
- Screening, i.e. mammography
- Self-examination
- Women with a mother, sister or daughter diagnosed with breast cancer have an 80% higher risk of being diagnosed with breast cancer themselves
- Having a first baby after age 30 or never having a baby

(Cancer Research UK 2008; Centre for Chronic Disease Prevention and Control 2007; Greenhalgh & Selfe 2006)

Age/gender

- 80% of cases are diagnosed after age 50 (Edith)
- More than 99% of breast cancer occurs in women (Edith)
- Up to 85% of women with breast cancer develop skeletal metastases before death

(Centre for Chronic Disease Prevention and Control 2007; White & Punjabi 1988)

Previous medical history

- Early menstruation (before age 12)
- Late menopause (after age 55)

(Cancer Research UK 2008; Centre for Chronic
Disease Prevention and Control 2007)

Lifestyle/environment/geography

- The highest rates of breast cancer occur in northern
  Europe (Edith) and North America and the lowest
  rates are in parts of Africa and Asia.
- Obesity increases risk of postmenopausal breast
  cancer by up to 30%.
- Women using hormone replacement therapy (HRT)
  for five years or longer have a 35% increased risk of
  breast cancer. In the UK, HRT causes an estimated
  2000 cases of breast cancer each year.
- The risk of breast cancer in current users of oral
  contraceptives is increased by around 25%.
- Drinking as little as one pint of beer or one glass of
  wine a day increases risk of breast cancer by more
  than 7%.
- A more active lifestyle reduces all cancer risk,
  including breast cancer.
- Women who smoked for >20 years have a 60%
  increase in the incidence of breast cancer.
- In women who smoke >20 cigarettes per day for 40
  years, the incidence rises to 83%.

(Cancer Research UK 2008; Centre for Chronic
Disease Prevention and Control 2007;
Terry et al 2002)

Objective examination

- 90% – lump
- 20% – painful lump
- 10% – nipple change
- 3% – nipple discharge
- 5% – skin contour change

Red Herrings

- Diffuse nodularity; common in all ages up to 50 years
- Cysts; peak age range 40–60 years

Differential diagnosis

- Fibroadenoma: peak age range 20–30 years
- Breast pain; pain alone is a very uncommon presentation of breast cancer

Gold standard investigations

'The ability to detect cancer at its very early stages when the patient is asymptomatic is the goal of every healthcare system'

(Kumar & Clark 2005)

Most common cancers start as focal microscopic clones of transformed cells and diagnosis only becomes likely once sufficient tumour bulk has accumulated to cause symptoms or signs. Screening processes are continually being developed to identify diseases at the earliest possible stage (National Cancer Institute 2008; Stephan 2007):

- Mammogram is the gold standard for breast cancer screening and early detection. Mammography can help detect 85–90% of all breast cancers, even before a lump is palpable.
- Biopsy

Pathology

Clinicians should be aware that one mechanism behind the distribution of metastatic disease is via tumour emboli entering the blood stream. In breast cancer, venous drainage from the breast via the azygos veins into the thoracic paravertebral venous plexus commonly leads to thoracic region metastases (Frymoyer 1997).

Timeline/prognosis (breast cancer)

The estimated relative five-year survival rate for women diagnosed as having breast cancer in England and Wales in 2001–2003 was 80%.
(Cancer Research UK 2008; West of Scotland Cancer Network 2006)

Evidence-based treatment

This depends on the stage of the disease but four types of standard treatment are employed (National Cancer Institute 2008):

- Surgery
- Radiotherapy
- Chemotherapy
- Hormone therapy

MALIGNANT SPINAL CORD COMPRESSION

Metastatic disease is the most common presentation for cancer in the spine; this can lead to malignant spinal cord compression (MSCC). Approximately 5% of all patients with cancer present with MSCC (Levack et al 2002). This would mean around 4000 cases per year in England and Wales or more than 100 cases per cancer network per year (NICE 2008). Levack et al (2002) emphasize that most patients with MSCC present initially to primary care clinicians with pain. In their study, MSCC was the first recorded symptom in 23% (n = 72) of patients presenting to a primary care clinic who were later diagnosed with cancer (Levack et al 2002).

Subjective examination

- Pain is almost always the first presenting symptom (Edith).
- Pain can start off as mild but escalates out of control despite analgesia (Edith).
- There is constant, progressive, severe pain in 84% of cases (Edith). The median visual analogue scale score is 8/10; 29% recorded pain as 'the worst imagined', 10/10, and in some cases 11/10 (Levack et al 2002).

- Pain is often associated with raised anxiety in the patient (Edith).
- New pain, or described as different to existing long-standing pain.
- Pain can be referred around the abdomen or chest in a band-like manner (Edith), often bilateral (66% of cases). These patients commonly describe a feeling of being squeezed.
- Pain is usually described as located in the back but radicular pain can be caused by Valsalva's manoeuvre, e.g. straining and coughing.
- Pain is described as: sharp (59%); shooting (41%); deep (36%).
- Pain may be aggravated by lying down (19%) (Edith). Bone pain is sometimes lesser if lying prone.
- Night pain.
- Pain may be eased by sitting.
- Thoracic pain should be treated as significant; it should not be assumed to be degenerative disc disease (Edith).
- Nerve pain in upper thighs.

(Christie Hospital NHS Foundation Trust 2007;
Greenhalgh & Selfe 2008;
Levack et al 2002;
West of Scotland Cancer Network 2006)

Clinically it is important to note that there can be a large discrepancy between site of pain and level of cord compression; these discrepancies can also be true for sensory deficit (Levack et al 2002).

Age/gender

- Highest prevalence – 40–65 years
- 89% patients over 50 years old (Edith)
- Men are less likely to consult for medical advice and therefore often present late

(Levack et al 2002; West of Scotland Cancer Network 2006)

Previous medical history

Patients with cancer who describe severe back or spinal root pain require urgent assessment (Edith) (Levack et al 2002).

Lifestyle/environment/geography

- Accessibility to healthcare – patients in remote communities often report later in the disease process
- Social norms may play a role in communities where there is low social acceptability of going to the doctor or where there is a predominantly fatalistic attitude that 'nothing can be done anyway'
- Smoking
- Alcohol
- Iatrogenic – e.g. alkylating agents, oestrogens, androgens and radiotherapy
- Diet – high fat intake
- Substance exposure, e.g. asbestos, vinyl chloride
- Ultraviolet radiation
- Biological agents, e.g. hepatitis B and C viruses

(Kumar & Clark 2005)

History of current episode

- Altered sensations in the legs
- Heaviness in the legs often associated with muscle weakness
- Prior to heaviness, patients may report their legs feel odd or strange

The following quote from our recent study with palliative care clinicians working in a hospice illustrates the clinical picture of altered leg sensations very well.

> 'The early ones usually say that their legs misbehave somehow, that they won't do what they want them to do. Their legs won't behave themselves, but they often won't present with that until it becomes more severe because they can't explain, or they're not sure, or don't know the significance of the fact that their legs are not doing what they want them to do. So finding their foot drops a little bit, or their right leg drags a bit they don't know the importance of that until much more serious symptoms and signs have actually developed.'

> (Greenhalgh & Selfe 2008)

Mobility and the ability to walk at the time of diagnosis of MSCC have been identified as key factors in improving the chance of maintaining independence as the disease progresses over time. Levack et al (2002) reported that only 18% of patients were able to walk at the time of diagnosis. Once the ability to walk has been lost, recovery of mobility is unlikely and many patients subsequently require nursing care (Edith). Lower limb weakness, and associated neurological deficit, are commonly recognized signs of cord compression which assist in the identification of the disease. Unfortunately, these findings are late manifestations of MSCC, therefore if clinicians suspect MSCC, urgent referral is needed (Levack et al 2002).

Objective examination

- Neurological deficit often occurs later in the disease process.
- Muscle weakness can begin in the lower limbs regardless of the level of cord compression.
- Difficulty in mobility, such as climbing stairs, reported falls, difficulty walking; interestingly, there appears no correlation between severity of pain and extent of neurological deficit.
- Compression at thoracic or cervical levels can result in upper limb weakness.
- L'hermitte's sign may be present with a tingling/shock-like sensation passing down the arms or trunk when the neck is flexed.
- Autonomic dysfunction such as constipation and/or retention along with ataxic gait and uncoordinated movements are usually late presenting symptoms.
- The thoracic spine is the commonest site of MSCC (68%) (Edith), followed by the lumbar (21%), cervical (7%), sacral (4%).

(Christie Hospital NHS Foundation Trust 2007; Greenhalgh & Selfe 2008; Levack et al 2002; West of Scotland Cancer Network 2006)

Red Herrings

- Chronic fatigue syndrome (ME)
- Fibromyalgia
- Widespread pain systems dysfunction
- Temporary improvement with conservative treatment
- Metabolic disorders

Differential diagnosis

- Upper motor neurone disease
- Multiple sclerosis
- Diabetes
- Alcoholism
- Cervical myopathy
- Peripheral neuropathy
- Lower limb oedema leading to heaviness in legs as a result of cardiovascular disease

Gold standard investigations

- Urgent (within 24 hours): magnetic resonance imaging (MRI) of the whole spine to confirm diagnosis, especially for those of known malignancy
- Full blood count (FBC), ESR, C-reactive protein (CRP) and biochemical profile, including urea and electrolytes (U&Es), liver function tests (LFTs), bone, and in men prostate-specific antigen (PSA)
- Immunoglobulins

- Urinalysis for Bence Jones proteins
- Chest X-ray, prostate or breast examination (to identify primary cancer)

(Levack et al 2002)

Delay in diagnosis and treatment can result in paraplegia (Edith) or quadriplegia depending on the site of the lesion, with a huge impact on quality of life and survival rate. Any patient suspected of having cord compression must be managed on an urgent basis.

Pathology

When metastases affect vertebral bone, the subsequent pathological fracture can result in compression of the cord, cauda equina or nerve roots with the possibility of subsequent paraplegia. Alternatively, the cord may be at risk from a soft tissue tumour. Multiple studies have consistently identified that diagnosis of MSCC frequently occurs late in the disease process with devastating consequences on the outcome of the patient (Levack et al 2002).

Timeline/prognosis (MSCC)

 The West of Scotland Guidelines (West of Scotland Cancer Network 2006) describe MSCC as presenting a median of six to eight weeks after the onset of the new back pain symptoms. Levack et al (2002) found that 94% of cases presenting with MSCC had pain, and that the pain had been present for approximately three months before a definitive diagnosis was given. From the point at which the patient first reported their relevant symptoms to a health professional, the mean time was two months. Most patients had reported their pain to a primary care clinician within three weeks.

Levack et al (2002) also report that patients with a previous diagnosis of cancer were diagnosed significantly more quickly than those with no prior diagnosis. Interestingly, the rate of diagnosis increased throughout the week to a maximum rate of diagnosis on a Friday. Of the six patients with cauda equina syndrome presenting to the Bolton Clinical Assessment, Treatment and Support (CATS) service in 2006, the majority were on a Friday. This apparently odd coincidence does not seem to be uncommon in clinical practice; it may be explained by patients' behaviour or alternatively it may be a feature of the way services are designed, however, to our knowledge, no clear explanation can be given.

Evidence-based treatment

Palliative radiotherapy is the commonest treatment in patients with MSCC. The aim of treatment is to reduce tumour size, relieve pain, and prevent progression of neurological deficit and recurrence. Radiotherapy is considered where there is a confirmed diagnosis of metastases and:

- The patient is unfit for surgery
- There is extensive vertebral involvement
- Multi-level disease is present

- The tumour is radiotherapy responsive, e.g. myeloma
- To prevent loss of sphincter control

(Christie Hospital NHS Foundation Trust 2007)

Surgical decompression and stabilization of the spine can improve outcome and reduce morbidity in selected cases. Early surgery, before severe neurological deficit, produces the best results and has less risk of wound complications if carried out prior to radiotherapy. Surgery is considered when:

- No diagnosis has been made
- Limited levels of cord compression are identified on imaging
- There is mild neurological impairment
- General health is suitable for general anaesthesia
- Life expectancy >6 months

Chemotherapy is limited in patients with MSCC to those with chemosensitive tumours (Christie Hospital NHS Foundation Trust 2007).

Summary

The medical evaluation of patients with spinal metastases is more complex than for those with isolated malignancies. A detailed clinical examination is essential in these cases to evaluate the extent of the illness (Rothman & Simeone 1992). According to Frymoyer (1997), any history of a known primary cancer, however remote, should be considered significant.

MYELOMA (PRIMARY DISEASE)

CASE 2: ANNIE

Annie, a 71-year-old woman, was seen by a CATS service with what appeared to be a resolving episode of sciatica. She had been attending an osteopath and her leg pain had resolved after six weeks. She still felt pain in the back and slightly towards the right side, however she was exercising. She was also sleeping most of the night although she did report some tossing and turning towards the end of the night. She found that bending and walking quickly as well as slump in sitting aggravated her symptoms but she was otherwise a fairly well woman, as described in the GP referral letter. At the time of attendance, she led an active life but had to slow down slightly due to her condition. She did report some weight loss, approximately 3 kg (6% of body weight) in the previous month, which she attributed to a reduced appetite due to pain.

 What are you thinking now?
What is your index of suspicion?

On examination she stood with what appeared to be a shift in the lumbar spine. This obviously created an asymmetry in her spine which the clinician felt may well be contributing to the mechanical stresses; however, Annie felt that this was a long-standing deformity since adolescence. There were no neurological symptoms or signs. She had reduced range of movement in her lumbar spine, especially extension. These findings were consistent with degenerative changes and would be unremarkable in view of her age.

She had appeared to have responded well to manual treatment and had followed the advice given to her. She had managed her episode of low back pain extremely well independently and was, at that point, improving. In the light of the improvement, the clinician explained to her that really there was very little else that could be done at that stage other than to continue with her exercises and give it some more time. A telephone review appointment was offered four weeks later, after Annie's imminent overseas summer holiday. Annie had some concerns about the length of the flight and her back pain.

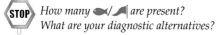

How many ⚑/⚑ are present?
What are your diagnostic alternatives?

Four weeks later, at the time of the telephone review, Annie revealed that she had been diagnosed with myeloma by her GP. A routine blood test performed at the practice in line with practice protocols had identified positive findings on protein electrophoresis.

CASE 3: BASIL

Basil was a pleasant, retired 65-year-old teacher who was referred for an orthopaedic opinion and was seen in a CATS service in August 2006. He had suffered from intermittent bouts of low back pain over many years. In recent years he had become aware of increasing episodes of low back pain that had begun to reduce his mobility. Over the last four months there had been a gradual deterioration in his symptoms with increasing right-sided low back pain and an onset of right lower leg pain in the L5 dermatome. He had been seen by an orthopaedic surgeon five years previously for one of these episodes and was treated with foot orthotics. X-rays arranged in August 2005 confirmed evidence of osteoarthritic change within the right hip and evidence of some subchondral sclerosis. Through his younger years, Basil had been very sporty, and regularly swam and played rugby. In his later years he had been a keen fell walker, although he had not been able to pursue this activity for several years due to his back pain.

On examination he was mobile with a stick and looked fairly well. He had a slightly stooped posture. There was a marked loss of lumbar lordosis and a slight increase in the thoracic kyphosis. There was virtually no lumbar extension and Basil complained of an increase in back pain at this point in the assessment. Left and right side flexion were moderately restricted. Flexion was relatively well preserved. Dural stress in a forward flexed position was negative. Sacro-iliac joint examination was normal. There was no power or sensory deficit, and reflexes, including the plantar response, were normal. The left hip had a well-preserved, pain-free range of movement. The right hip had a very slight restriction to movement, which was pain free but was considered to display an excellent range of movement for his age. He had no weight loss and he was systemically well.

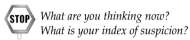

What are you thinking now?
What is your index of suspicion?

The history and examination findings were thought by the clinician to be suggestive of degenerative disc disease with associated central and lateral recess stenosis that had resulted in a right L5 nerve root irritation. However, in view of his age and progressively worsening leg symptoms, the clinician thought it was prudent to arrange blood tests to exclude underlying pathology and an MRI scan.

 How many 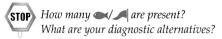 are present?
What are your diagnostic alternatives?

The results of Basil's initial blood tests identified a high ESR of 68 mm/h. A previous ESR in 2002 was 14 mm/h (normal reported range 4–10 mm/h). It was noted his urea was high at 10.5 mmol/L (normal reported range 2.8–7.2 mmol/L), creatinine high at 129 µmol/L (normal reported range 62–124 µmol/L) and haemoglobin low at 12.5 g/dL (normal reported range 13–18 g/dL). A previous haemoglobin test result in March 2005 was 17 g/dL. In view of these results the MRI was expedited.

 What are you thinking now?

The presentation was of worsening mild renal failure and mild anaemia combined with a high ESR. The most likely diagnosis was multiple myeloma. A repeat ESR, repeat FBC and protein electrophoresis were organized. The results of his repeat ESR showed a further rise to 104 mm/h.

 What are you going to do next?

An urgent referral and communication with secondary care haematology took place.

The MRI identified diffuse marrow infiltration consistent with suspected multiple myeloma, although there was evidence of compression of the right L4 nerve root by disc herniation. Multiple myeloma was later confirmed by the haematology department. Sadly Basil died after only four months from presenting to the service.

MULTIPLE MYELOMA

Myeloma is the only primary malignant spinal cancer. Other cancers that occur in the spine are due to secondary infiltration of metastases. Multiple myeloma is not curable, however early diagnosis reduces the risks of progressive spinal cord compression (UK Myeloma Forum 2006). Every year in the UK, almost 3800 cases of multiple myeloma are diagnosed, and the condition causes more than 2400 deaths in the UK each year (Cancer Research UK 2007).

Subjective examination

Subjective examination gives clearer indications of serious pathology than objective findings. The clinical history plays a greater role in the early stages of the disease; objective physical examination is more informative in later stages of disease (Chorti, personal communication 2007; Deyo et al 1992).

Age/gender

- Increasing age is the most significant risk factor for multiple myeloma.
- 95% of cases of myeloma are diagnosed after age 50 (Annie, Basil).
- Average age of onset is 65 (Basil).
- Males are twice as likely to develop myeloma compared to females (Basil).

(American Cancer Association 2005; Department of Health 2000; UK Myeloma Forum 2006)

Previous medical history

- Multiple myeloma seems to be more common in some families. If a person has a sibling or parent with myeloma, their chance of developing it is nearly four times that of the general population.

(American Cancer Association 2005)

Lifestyle/environment/geography

- Being overweight or obese increases a person's risk of developing myeloma.
- Multiple myeloma is more than twice as common among black Americans as among white Americans.
- Workers in petroleum-related industries may be at higher risk.

(American Cancer Association 2005)

History of current episode

- Myeloma can remain dormant for as long as three years.

- The prodromal phase can last between five and 20 years.
- The most common presentation of multiple myeloma is bone pain particularly in the back. This is commonly associated with lower limb radiculopathy; there may also be associated fractures.
- The intensity of pain seems greater than in other conditions, with a more searing quality and more constant, not affected by movement.

(Department of Health 2000; Deyo et al 1992; Goodman et al 1998; Greenhalgh & Selfe 2006, 2008; International Myeloma Foundation 2002)

Objective examination

- Bone destruction, i.e. loss of height, especially in men and pre-menopausal women
- Spinal cord and nerve root compression
- Recurrent/persistent bacterial infection
- Anaemia (Basil)
- Persistent elevation of ESR or plasma viscosity (Basil)
- Hypercalcaemia
- Impaired renal function (Basil)

(Department of Health 2000; UK Myeloma Forum 2006)

Red Herrings

- Temporary improvement with conservative treatment (Annie).

Bone scans can be negative in myeloma due to impaired osteoblastic activity. The bone scan will not become positive until a fracture has occurred; consequently bone scanning is not usually helpful in the diagnosis of myeloma.

(UK Myeloma Forum 2006)

Differential diagnosis

- Simple mechanical low back pain
- Nerve root entrapment
- Malignant cord compression from another cause

Gold standard investigations

- X-rays are the gold standard investigation for myeloma. A full skeletal survey for myeloma using a series of X-rays is needed to identify bone destruction, lytic lesions, and/or any fracture or collapse of bone.
- MRI is used when X-rays are negative yet serious pathology is still suspected, for more detailed testing of the spine. MRI scans have a 0.95 sensitivity for identifying focal bone marrow lesions. In practice, this may be the first radiological investigation to confirm a cause for concern, initiating the skeletal survey.
- MRI is also very useful for quantifying the degree of cord compression.
- MRI can also identify disease in soft tissue, which may be compromising nerve roots and/or the spinal cord.

- Bone marrow biopsy confirms presence of malignant cells in the bone marrow. This is the most important test to establish the percentage of myeloma cells in the bone marrow. In solitary plasmacytoma, biopsy of the tumour mass itself is performed.
- A full blood count should be performed to:
  - Identify presence and severity of anaemia
  - Identify low white cell count
  - Identify low blood platelet count.
- U&Es are especially important to investigate kidney function and for calcium levels.

(Dimopoulos et al 2000; Liebross et al 1998; UK Myeloma Forum 2006) (Table 5.1).

Table 5.1 Interpretation of results of tests in myeloma (UK Myeloma Forum 2006)

Test	Myeloma
Bone marrow plasma cells	>10% on aspirate
Serum paraprotein	Variable concentration in serum; no specific diagnostic levels
Bence Jones proteinuria	>50% cases
Immune paresis	>95% cases
Lytic bone lesions	Often present
Anaemia	Frequent
Hypercalcaemia	May be present
Abnormal renal function	May be present

Pathology

Malignant myeloma is a primary malignant bone tumour which develops from excessive plasma cell growth in the bone marrow. The proliferation of plasma cells causes an excessive stimulation of osteoclastic activity resulting in bone reabsorption. The rise in osteoclast activity is not matched by a corresponding increase in osteoblastic activity, therefore one of the features of multiple myeloma is osteoporosis.

In addition, the overgrowth of plasma cells can interfere with the normal blood-forming functions of the bone marrow, resulting in a shortage of red blood cells, leading to anaemia and fatigue. A shortage of platelets can also occur; this can cause problems with clotting leading to excessive bleeding after cuts. Another problem caused by an excess of plasma cells is leucopenia, where there is a shortage of white blood cells, which can reduce resistance to infections (American Cancer Association 2005).

Timeline/prognosis (multiple myeloma)

- The median survival varies from 7.5 to 12 years Adverse prognostic features include older age and larger lesions (Basil)
- A negative MRI of the spine is a good prognostic feature

(Dimopoulos et al 2000;
Liebross et al 1998)

Evidence-based treatment

- A consultant haematologist or oncologist should lead the care of patients with multiple myeloma.
- Proteasome inhibitors slow myeloma cell growth.
- Bisphosphonates maintain bone health.
- Localized bone lesions can be treated with radiotherapy.
- Exercise therapy maintains bone density and reduces the effects of fatigue during radiotherapy and chemotherapy. Exercises need careful prescription in order to avoid overload leading to pathological fractures.

(Coon & Coleman 2004; UK Myeloma Forum 2006)

SUMMARY

These three cases illustrate the challenges that face clinicians in diagnosing spinal malignancy. This challenge is even greater early in the disease process. The clinician must reach a balance between not over-investigating the 'worried well' and not missing serious cases such as these. Edith presented at a much later stage in the disease process than Annie and Basil and yet the case highlights the difficulty clinicians face. Each year, medical practice becomes more efficient at identifying these diseases much earlier in their natural history; the use of screening mammograms for the identification of breast cancer, which began in the 1980s, is a good example. The development of awareness, vigilance and suspicion within clinicians, supported by scientific advancement, will continue to improve the early detection rates of cancer.

References

Abbott M, Lefton D, Abbott R et al 2003 Osteoblastoma. Paediatric Neurosurgery 39: 279–281

American Cancer Association 2005 Multiple myeloma. Online. Available: www.cancer.org/docroot/lrn/lrn_0.asp (accessed 2 July 2008)

Australian Department of Health and Ageing 2004 Cancer data and trends. Online. Available: http://www.health.gov.au (accessed 3 August 2004)

Cancer Research UK 2007 Multiple myeloma. Online. Available: http://info.cancerresearchuk.org/cancerstats/types/multiplemyeloma/?a=5441 (accessed 12 June 2008)

Cancer Research UK 2008 Cancer statistics. Online. Available: http://info.cancerresearchuk.org/cancerstats (accessed 12 May 2008)

Centre for Chronic Disease Prevention and Control 2007 Breast cancer. Online. Available: http://www.phac-aspc.gc.ca (accessed 12 May 2008)

Christie Hospital NHS Foundation Trust 2007 Spinal cord compression guidelines. Christie Hospital, Manchester

Coon S K, Coleman E A 2004 Keep moving: patients with myeloma talk about exercise and fatigue. Oncology Nursing Forum 31: 1127–1135

Department of Health 2000 Referral guidelines for suspected cancer. Department of Health, London

Deyo R A, Rainville J, Kent D L 1992 What can the history and physical examination tell us about low back pain? Journal of the American Medical Association 268: 760–765

Dimopoulos M A, Moulopoulos L A, Maniatis A et al 2000 Solitary plasmacytoma of bone and asymptomatic multiple myeloma. Blood 96: 2037–2044

European Commission 2004 Health statistics. Key data on health 2002 (data 1970–2001). European Commission

Frymoyer J W 1997 The adult spine: principles and practice, 2nd edn. Lippincott-Raven, Philadelphia

Goodman C C, Fuller K S, Boissonnault W G 1998 Pathology implications for physical therapists, 2nd edn. W B Saunders, Philadelphia

Greenhalgh S, Selfe J 2004 Margaret: a tragic case of spinal Red Flags and Red Herrings. Physiotherapy 90: 73–76

Greenhalgh S, Selfe J 2006 Red Flags: a guide to identifying serious pathology of the spine, 1st edn. Churchill Livingstone, Elsevier, Edinburgh

Greenhalgh S, Selfe J 2008 Red Flags for serious spinal pathology: a qualitative study of palliative care clinicians' opinion. Chartered Society of Physiotherapy, Annual Congress, Manchester

International Myeloma Foundation 2002 Patient handbook. International Myeloma Foundation, Edinburgh

Kumar P, Clark M 2005 Clinical medicine, 6th edn. W B Saunders, Edinburgh

Levack P, Graham J, Collie D et al 2002 Don't wait for a sensory level – listen to the symptoms: a prospective audit of the delays in diagnosis of malignant cord compression. Clinical Oncology 14: 472–480

Liebross R H, Ha C S, Cox J D et al 1998 Solitary bone plasmacytoma: outcome and prognostic factors following radiotherapy. International Journal of Radiation, Oncology, Biology, Physics 41: 1063–1067

National Cancer Institute 2008 Breast cancer treatment. Online. Available: www.cancer.gov/cancertopics/pdq/treatment/breast/Patient#Keypoint4 (accessed 15 July 2008)

National Institute for Health and Clinical Excellence 2008 Metastatic spinal cord compression: diagnosis and management of adults at risk of and with metastatic spinal cord compression. Clinical guideline 75. Online. Available: www.nice.org.uk/Guidance/CG75 (accessed 3 February 2009)

Rothman R H, Simeone F A 1992 The spine, 3rd edn. W B
    Saunders, Edinburgh
Stephan P 2007 Diagnosis of breast cancer. Online. Available:
    http://breastcancer.about.com/od/diagnosis/a/diagnosis_
    ov.htm (accessed 15 July 2008)
Terry P D, Miller A B, Rohan T E 2002 Cigarette smoking and
    breast cancer: a long latency period. International Journal of
    Cancer 100: 723–728
UK Myeloma Forum 2006 Myeloma. Online. Available: www.
    ukmf.org.uk (accessed 16 November 2006)
West of Scotland Cancer Network 2006 West of Scotland
    guidelines for malignant spinal cord compression. West of
    Scotland Cancer Network
White A A, Punjabi M M 1988 Biomechanical considerations in
    the surgical management of cervical spondylitic myelopathy.
    Spine 13: 856–860
WHO 2004 Cancer. Online. Available: www.who.int/cancer
    (accessed 22 April 2004)

Chapter 6

Serious Pathology Fractures

THREE CASES OF SERIOUS PATHOLOGY FRACTURES

CASE 1: ETHEL

Ethel was a pleasant 76-year-old woman who was referred for an orthopaedic opinion via a clinical specialist from an accident and emergency department (A&E). Ethel had suffered a fall in January 2007, when she tripped forwards and landed heavily onto the right side of her body, injuring the right side of her face and fracturing two fingers. She was immediately aware of low back pain, which persisted for the months following her injury. She was managing this pain with some difficulty and six weeks previously she had suffered an onset of acute right-sided back, buttock, groin and leg pain, which resulted in an attendance at A&E. She was admitted for two days and underwent X-rays, which showed no fracture and no bony abnormality. Despite some improvement she still complained of localized discomfort at the base of her lumbar spine into the right buttock, intermittently into the right groin and into the right antero-medial thigh and upper lateral aspect of the right leg. She had no anaesthesia or paraesthesia. Bladder and bowel functions were normal. Symptoms tended to be aggravated by prolonged periods of bending, stooping or walking; her sleep was not disturbed. Ethel reported good health; she was a non-smoker and drank little alcohol. It was documented that she was on medication for hypertension and was taking paracetamol for pain relief.

On examination it was noted she was independently mobile with a slightly rolling gait. No spinal deviations were present. The lumbar spine had minimal equal restriction on all movements which increased general low back discomfort. Sacro-iliac joint examination was normal. The right hip had full passive movement with significant end range tightness and buttock pain, particularly on rotations and flexion; resisted hip tests were pain free. Ethel had no neurological signs or symptoms, and all nerve tests were recorded as normal. There was marked tenderness localized to the right sacro-iliac joint and deep in the right buttock along the line of the piriformis muscle.

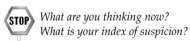

What are you thinking now?
What is your index of suspicion?

The clinician reviewed her X-ray and the accompanying report and concluded that no fracture or bony abnormality was evident. The clinician also reviewed her blood test results, which showed normal C-reactive protein (CRP) levels/thyroid function/bone profile and an erythrocyte sedimentation rate (ESR) of 25 mm/h (normal reported range 4–10 mm/h). It was noted however, that her previous ESR, one month earlier, was 18 mm/h. The clinician felt that the findings were consistent with

> '(R) sacro-iliac joint dysfunction with a possible right L5 root irritation.'

The clinician felt that there was no indication for further orthopaedic investigation or management at that time and a recently started course of physiotherapy should continue with an orthopaedic review if necessary.

Ethel was concurrently referred to a member of the Clinical Assessment, Treatment and Support (CATS) service team for advice on pain management. This was carried out by a supplementary prescriber who conducted a detailed drugs history as part of the consultation. At this consultation her leg pain had settled and her symptoms were localized to low back pain. Subjective questioning revealed that she had a family history of osteoporosis. She had also been told more than 20 years ago by the family general practitioner (GP) that she potentially had osteoporosis and had been treated with Didronel (a bisphosphonate).

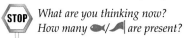

STOP *What are you thinking now?*
How many ⬛/◢ are present?

At the time of this attendance, although Ethel's leg pain had improved, her low back pain was out of control and Ethel also described a loss of height. This was confirmed on examination as her actual height was around 5 cm less than her reported height.

 What are your diagnostic alternatives?

In view of the uncontrolled pain, a magnetic resonance imaging (MRI) scan was organized. This revealed an old wedge compression fracture of the body at the level of T12. Ethel was shown her MRI findings and, interestingly, to some degree she felt reassured that something had been found, despite this level being completely pain free. Importantly, this 'positive' finding was distant from the site of pain. There was no obvious irritation of the L5 nerve root on the image at the time of this attendance. The wedge fracture of T12 was, however, potentially diagnostic of osteoporosis.

 What will you do next with this patient?

Ethel was referred to the bone health team at the local primary care trust for an up-to-date bone health screen and drug review to assist her pain management.

 What is challenging about this case?

CASE 2: ERIC

In April 2004, Eric presented to an orthopaedic triage service following referral from his GP. Eric was a 56-year-old retired taxi driver, who was disabled due to Parkinson's disease, which began six years previously and for which he was under the care of the consultant neurologists at the local district general hospital. Until the end of 2003, Eric was fairly active and able to walk with a stick and ride his bike. Eric chose to stand in the waiting room prior to the consultation and throughout the consultation itself due to an exacerbation of symptoms on sitting. Eric described a history of a fall from his bike onto his right hip at the beginning of November. He got back on to the bike but felt pain immediately, extending into the right abdominal area. By the next morning he had developed severe right leg pain and experienced difficulty putting weight on to that leg. Prior to his attendance in late spring, physiotherapy had been attempted and treatment included mobilization/manipulation, hydrotherapy and electrotherapy; in addition, Eric had consulted a private physiotherapist. Despite this variety of physiotherapy interventions, Eric felt that his right leg had become gradually weaker since the accident.

 What are you thinking now?
What is your index of suspicion?

When Eric arrived for his appointment he needed to walk with a frame and relied very heavily on this for support. He was unable to sit at all due to the acute pain in the right buttock and leg. Eric described his right posterior thigh as 'feeling woolly'; he found this woolly sensation in the posterior thigh very difficult to tolerate. A form of allodynia had also developed in the right foot with the lateral aspect of the foot feeling numb. As a consequence Eric needed to wear three pairs of socks, partly to keep his foot warm, but partly to cushion the sole of his foot from discomfort during weight bearing.

He described some partial saddle anaesthesia, particularly on the right side, but no disturbance with bladder or bowel function. A cough and sneeze were negative.

STOP *What are you thinking now?*

Eric described his pain as present 24 hours a day. This no longer appeared mechanical in nature and was described by the clinician in a clinic letter as

'having a very sinister character to it'.

As described earlier, sitting made his symptoms much worse and nothing helped to relieve his pain. Eric's sleep was only disturbed slightly. First thing in the morning he had great difficulty getting going, particularly moving his right leg. In general, however, he felt well and his weight was stable, although he was concerned about the significant deterioration in his mobility.

STOP *How many* *are present?*

An MRI of the lumbar spine had been arranged by his consultant neurologist, and at the time of his attendance Eric was waiting for that appointment.

On examination, Eric's gait was very poor and he relied heavily on the frame for support. He was unable to sit at all and stood throughout the subjective questioning, as he did waiting for the appointment, but there was no evidence of any pain system dysfunction or abnormal illness behaviour. His movements in standing revealed very poor core stability, but it was difficult to establish how much of this was due to his Parkinson's

disease at that first appointment. Actual spinal movements could not be carried out effectively as Eric
needed such a lot of support from the frame, but spinal
movements with support from the clinician and the
walking frame did not increase his leg pain. With some
difficulty Eric managed to lie on the examination couch
for further examination. He had tight hamstrings both
on the left and the right, but interestingly straight leg
raise did not provoke his right leg pain. He had marked
right-sided weakness of the peronei, with weakness also
of extensor hallucis and tibialis anterior to a lesser
degree. Eric had numbness of the lateral aspect of the
right foot in the S1 dermatome and his right ankle jerk
was absent. In addition, there was some slight saddle
anaesthesia. Rectal examination revealed weakness of
his anal sphincter and sensory blunting on the right side
of the perineum. The body of the sacrum was very
tender as was the right pelvic wall. It was interesting to
find that he was acutely tender around the right sacral
notch and right buttock, which reproduced his symptoms down the right leg to the foot. However, palpation
of the spine was unremarkable.

 What are your diagnostic alternatives?

An X-ray of both hips and pelvis was arranged
which was later reported as negative. An MRI was
therefore organized. The MRI identified degenerative
changes in the lower lumbar spine, but it also appeared
to show what was described by the radiologist as

'a new infiltrative lesion in the right half of the sacrum'.

This was suggestive of serious pathology. There did not appear to be any bony destruction and no obvious soft tissue mass, but the MRI report suggested that there did seem to be some degree of reaction in the soft tissues around the sacrum. This would suggest some type of inflammatory activity within the soft tissues.

 What will you do next with this patient?

An urgent computed tomography (CT) scan was organized to clarify what was going on in the bone.

 What is challenging about this case?
What assumptions have you made about this case ?
What is your level of plausibility and certainty?

The CT scan revealed evidence of a non-united vertical sheer fracture through the right half of the sacrum. The doctor who reported the films was convinced that this was a straightforward traumatic fracture with no evidence of underlying pathological abnormality, as there was no disruption of the anterior part of the pelvic ring. There was no evidence of compressive pathology in the spinal cord, either on the MRI or CT scan, but the fracture clearly involved the sacral foramina at the S1 and S2 levels.

CASE 3: DEREK

Derek was a 53-year-old retired postman who 12 months previously had been diagnosed with cirrhosis of the liver due to a genetic disorder. He had complained of episodes of low back pain on and off for years, however an episode of low back pain was exacerbated in December 2007 while carrying an empty fish tank. At the time of his attendance to an orthopaedic triage service his symptoms had deteriorated further. At the time of his appointment he was unable to control his pain well as he was intolerant of tramadol due to his liver cirrhosis. He was only able to tolerate paracetamol to a maximum of 2000 mg daily (this equates to half the maximum dose for an adult) but this was offering little relief. In addition he had also tried local heat, transcutaneous electric nerve stimulation (TENS) and analgesic sprays, without success.

Derek's main complaint was distinct severe pain in the lower lumbar region. There were no radicular signs, however pain was particularly sensitive to movement and was especially irritable. Sleep was not being disturbed to any great extent.

Examination revealed a reduced lumbar lordosis and minimal lumbar range of movement. Throughout range, pain increased especially on side flexion bilaterally. Straight leg raising and examination of the hips were both normal but Derek had tenderness bilaterally on the iliac crests. There were no specific neurological deficits in the lower limbs but there was bilateral ankle oedema. Lumbar palpation revealed nothing abnormal.

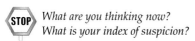

What are you thinking now?
What is your index of suspicion?

How many ⚫/◢ are present?
What will you do next with this patient?

In view of his presenting symptoms and medical history, Derek was referred for an MRI scan of his lumbar spine to exclude serious pathology.

 What is challenging about this case?
What are your diagnostic alternatives?

The MRI scan identified osteoporosis and multi-level compression fractures at L1–L5. These compression fractures were reported as appearing acute to subacute at L3–L5.

Following the initial orthopaedic triage assessment, Derek unfortunately fractured his hip. He described being nagged by his wife to help with the washing. As he was carrying the washing to the dryer, he tripped and fractured his neck of femur. It took Derek an hour to crawl to the phone to call for help and unfortunately the washing never made it into the dryer! Derek was under the care of the orthopaedic team at the local district general hospital when the MRI results were received. The clinicians involved in Derek's case were alerted to the MRI findings so that they could act accordingly.

 What assumptions have been made about this case ?

In Derek's case, his diagnosis of cirrhosis was as a consequence of a genetic problem. However, a common cause of cirrhosis is alcoholism.

OSTEOPOROSIS/FRACTURES

SUBJECTIVE EXAMINATION

- Fracture associated with minimal trauma (Derek)
- Falls history; number and mechanism; any associated injury (Ethel, Eric, Derek)
- Menopausal status including age at menopause and number of years since menopause (Ethel)
- Exercise status – past and current
- Any self-reported loss of height (Ethel)
- Difficulty lying in bed; any increase in number of pillows needed

(Bennell et al 2000)

Age/gender

- Osteoporosis can occur in all populations at all ages (Ethel, Derek)
- Most prevalent in post-menopausal Caucasian women (Ethel)
- In women over 60 it is estimated the lifetime risk of vertebral fracture is 1 in 3 (Ethel)

(National Institute for Health and Clinical Excellence (NICE) 2005)

The social and acute care costs of osteoporotic fractures in post-menopausal women in the UK are estimated to be in the region of £1030 million (NICE 2005).

Previous medical history

- Genetic disposition (Derek)
- Family history (Ethel)
- Mother who had a hip fracture before the age of 75
- Rheumatoid arthritis
- Amenorrhoea
- Chronic inflammatory bowel disease
- Hyperthyroidism
- Coeliac disease
- Corticosteroids
- Hormone replacement therapy (HRT)

(Bennell et al 2000; International Osteoporosis Foundation 2008; NICE 2005)

Lifestyle/environment/geography

- Alcoholism
- Smoking
- Low body mass index (BMI) of less than 19 kg/m²
- Low calcium diet
- Vitamin deficiency
- Prolonged immobilization

Approximately 99% of the total calcium in the body is contained in bone; most adults require at least 1000 mg/day of calcium, which can be obtained from dairy products and green leafy vegetables (International Osteoporosis Foundation 2008; NICE 2005; Niewoehner & Niewoehner 1999).

History of current episode

Many individuals are unaware that they have osteoporosis until they sustain a fracture (Derek) (Bennell et al 2000).

OBJECTIVE EXAMINATION

- Vertebral compression fractures can cause loss of height. This may occur suddenly or gradually over time (Ethel)
- Thoracic kyphosis (dowager's hump)
- The distance between the rib cage and the iliac crests can decrease and, if severe, pain may be experienced due to the lower ribs pressing on the pelvis. This may also lead to respiratory and digestive problems
- Postural changes may cause some patients to develop a 'pot belly' with concertina-like skin folds

(Bennell et al 2000)

RED HERRINGS

◄ Pain systems dysfunction

DIFFERENTIAL DIAGNOSIS

Any patient with a spinal fracture should be screened for serious pathology.

GOLD STANDARD INVESTIGATIONS

Osteoporosis is diagnosed by measuring bone mineral density with a scanner using dual energy X-ray absorptiometry (DEXA). The results are given as a T-score.

A T-score of within −1 SD of normal bone density is classed as normal. A T-score between −1 SD and −2.5 SD shows some bone weakness and a T-score below −2.5 SD is considered to show osteoporosis. Bone mineral density assessed by DEXA is also currently the best single predictor of the risk of future fracture of an individual. It is, most often, the only diagnostic tool available for clinicians in daily practice.

Once fracture has occurred, X-ray or CT would be the investigation of choice (NICE 2005).

PATHOLOGY

The balance between bone resorption and bone deposition is determined by osteoclasts and osteoblasts. Osteoclasts have highly active ion channels in the cell membrane that pump protons into the extracellular space; this lowers the pH which dissolves the bone mineral. In contrast, osteoblasts lay down new bone mineral. The balance between the activities of these two cell types governs whether bone is made, maintained or lost. In a normal bone remodelling cycle, osteoclasts are activated first, leading to bone resorption. Because the bone formation phase takes longer than the resorption phase, any increase in remodelling activity can result in an overall loss of bone (Niewoehner & Niewoehner 1999).

Hormones are possibly the most important modulators of bone formation. It is well established that oestrogen, parathyroid hormone and, to a lesser extent, testosterone are essential for healthy bone formation and maintenance. Oestrogen is believed to have the most direct effect on bone cells, interacting with specific receptors, on the surface of osteoblasts and osteoclasts. When oestrogen levels drop, bone turnover increases and an imbalance develops encouraging proportionately more bone resorption (International Osteoporosis Foundation 2008).

The effects of corticosteroids on bone loss are well known and are an important concern in patients who require systemic corticosteroid therapy for more than three months (Table 6.1). Corticosteroids inhibit calcium

Table 6.1 Effects of corticosteroids on bone metabolism (adapted from Niewoehner & Niewoehner 1999)

Decreased	Increased
Bone protein synthesis	Collagen degradation
Bone growth factors	Renal calcium excretion
Osteoblast number	Parathyroid hormone action
Intestinal calcium absorption	
Oestrogen and androgen production	

absorption across the intestine independent of vitamin D levels and increase renal calcium excretion, resulting in a negative calcium balance. This results in secondary hyperparathyroidism, which increases bone resorption.

The trabecular bone of the axial skeleton is particularly vulnerable to systemic corticosteroid therapy. The long-term use of corticosteroids can result in vertebral and rib fractures, which are often accompanied by back and chest wall pain. Anyone receiving frequent or prolonged (more than three months) systemic corticosteroid treatment is at increased risk for osteoporosis. There is no evidence to date that low doses of inhaled corticosteroids as used in the treatment of asthma have adverse effects on bones (Niewoehner & Niewoehner 1999).

Timeline/prognosis

- Postmenopausal bone loss can be as great as 5% per year.
- During the first six months of corticosteroid therapy, vertebral bone loss can be especially severe, with decreases of 6–10% in bone mineral density commonly occurring. Thereafter, the rate of loss slows to 1–2% per year, which is still two to three times the rate associated with normal ageing.

EVIDENCE-BASED TREATMENT

Pharmacology

Bisphosphonates are recommended by NICE (2005) (Ethel):

- Alendronate
- Etidronate
- Risedronate

Bisphosphonates prevent the breakdown of bone. Calcium supplements may also be used.

Exercise

The exact exercise dose required for maximal skeletal effects is not yet known, it is, however, recommended that exercise should be performed two to three times per week. For aerobic exercise, sessions should last between 15 and 60 minutes. The average conditioning intensity recommended for adults without fragility fractures is between 70% and 80% of their functional capacity. Periodic progression of exercise dosage is needed otherwise bone adaptation will cease. Increasing the intensity or weight bearing is more effective than increasing the duration of the exercise. When considering posture and flexibility in patients with osteopenia or osteoporosis, treatment should aim to minimize the flexion load on the spine, promote an extended posture and improve chest expansion (Bennell et al 2000).

In a randomized controlled trial of 53 women with spinal crush fracture and back pain, a 10-week physiotherapy programme, consisting of balance training, muscle strengthening and lumbar stabilization exercises, was effective in decreasing analgesic use and back pain and increasing quality of life and level of daily function (Malmros et al 1998).

The following management recommendations for patients with osteoporosis are drawn from the Chartered Society of Physiotherapy (CSP 1999) physiotherapy guidelines for the management of osteoporosis:

- Maintain bone strength
- Prevent fractures
- Improve muscle strength, balance, cardiovascular fitness
- Improve posture
- Improve psychological well-being
- Provide education
- Aim to reduce falls
- Exercise management for bone health
- Strength training

In an exercise regimen, it is advised that the overload principle is applied through a relatively high load and low repetitions regimen. Any form of strength training needs to be site specific, i.e. targeting areas such as the muscle groups around the hip, quadriceps, dorsi-plantar flexors, rhomboids, wrist extensors and back extensors. Weight-bearing exercises should be targeted to loading bone sites predominantly affected by osteoporotic change, i.e. hip, vertebrae and wrist. Exercise should be used in combination with both adequate calcium intake and some type of clinical therapy for maintaining and/or increasing bone mineral density. All exercise programmes should start at an easy level and be progressive in terms of intensity and impact.

Precautions

The following activities should be avoided (CSP 1999):

- High impact exercise
- Trunk flexion and lifting
- Trunk rotational torsion movements with any loading

SUMMARY

These three cases illustrate three very distinct precipitating factors leading to vertebral fracture, Ethel probably illustrating the more common type of fracture presentation in a primary care setting. The cases also illustrate the different radiological approaches to identifying specific aspects of bone pathology. A DEXA performed years earlier may well have alerted Ethel's GP to her risk of future fracture. Eric's subtle fracture was not clearly evident on MRI. CT was necessary to provide a clearer image of the bone, but MRI was adequate in Derek's case to reveal the cause of the pain. Clinical reasoning in spinal cases where fracture is a possibility must consider:

'Why might there be a fracture?'

- Is the bone health at risk for a known reason?
- Was the trauma of significant impact?
- Could there be an as yet unknown pathological cause?

Remember healthy spines do not just fracture!

References

Bennell K, Khan K, McKay H 2000 The role of physiotherapy in the prevention and treatment of osteoporosis. Manual Therapy 5: 198–213

Chartered Society of Physiotherapy 1999 Physiotherapy guidelines for the management of osteoporosis. Chartered Society of Physiotherapy, London

International Osteoporosis Foundation 2008 Osteoporosis. Online. Available: www.iofbonehealth.org/home.html (accessed 2 July 2008)

Malmros B, Mortenson L, Jensen M B et al 1998 Positive effects of physiotherapy on chronic pain and performance in osteoporosis. Osteoporosis International 8: 215–221

National Institute for Health and Clinical Excellence 2005 Prevention and treatment of osteoporosis. National Institute for Health and Clinical Excellence, London

Niewoehner C B, Niewoehner D E 1999 Steroid-induced osteoporosis. Are your asthmatic patients at risk? Postgraduate Medicine 105:79–83, 87–8, 91

Chapter 7

Red Herrings

CASE 1: GERALDINE

Geraldine presented to an outpatient clinic complaining of low back pain in 2003. She was a 55-year-old woman, married with a 23-year-old son and was also a carer for her mother, who had suffered several strokes. Her subjective history revealed that seven years previously, her initial problem was a numb left hand for which she consulted an orthopaedic surgeon. She went on to have nerve conduction studies which did not confirm carpal tunnel syndrome and so no further treatment was offered. At a similar time Geraldine remembered having a feeling

> *'like a guitar string vibrating'*

going down her back into the left leg; this was brought on by neck flexion.

 What are you thinking now?
What is your index of suspicion?

Geraldine was treated with a number of courses of physiotherapy without success. The numbness of the left hand never recovered and at some point, probably within the next year, she began to stumble with the left leg and felt that it was dragging when she walked any distance. This very slowly got worse over the years, with the leg just not quite feeling right. Geraldine reported a distinct feeling of altered sensation at the top of the thigh. At the time of presentation, Geraldine was able to walk for 15 minutes without stopping.

Geraldine had developed bladder disturbance in the form of a mild progressive urgency of micturition but she was not incontinent. Unlike her back pain, these bladder symptoms had not been severe enough to prompt her to seek medical attention.

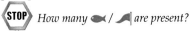 *How many* 🐟 / 🚩 *are present?*

On examination she had a good range of spinal movement; straight leg raise and femoral nerve stretch were unremarkable. However, there appeared to be a briskness of the reflexes in both the upper and lower limbs, more obvious on the left, and the plantar response was upward going. There was also a mild heel–shin ataxia on the left.

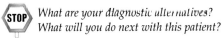 *What are your diagnostic alternatives?*
What will you do next with this patient?

A magnetic resonance imaging (MRI) scan of Geraldine's head and neck was organized, along with referral to a neurologist. The scan showed non-specific white matter lesions that were not particularly periventricular, but there was a spinal cord lesion in the dorsal part of the spinal cord at the mid-cervical level.

Geraldine was diagnosed by the neurologist as having a primary progressive multiple sclerosis (MS) and the MRI scan supported this diagnosis. Fortunately Geraldine's disease was relatively non-progressive, which was reassuring. Specific treatment options at the time of presentation were not available. The neurologist referred Geraldine to the MS nurse team and she was to be reviewed annually or as her condition dictated.

L'HERMITTE'S SIGN

L'hermitte's sign is provoked by cervical flexion and is highly suggestive of spinal cord involvement; it is most commonly described in the orthopaedic literature as:

'an electric shock like feeling which shoots down the spine and occasionally into the arms.'

L'hermitte's sign is a common sign of acute exacerbations of MS. Many authorities feel that the presence of this sign should immediately raise the suspicion of MS, but it can also occur in cases of:

- Cervical myelopathy
- Subacute combined degeneration of the spinal cord
- Radiation myelopathy
- Spinal cord compression

A reversed L'hermitte's sign is provoked by cervical extension; this is strongly associated with cervical spondylosis. Geraldine clearly described L'hermitte's sign but not in the textbook way outlined above:

'a feeling like a guitar string vibrating, going down my back into the left leg.'

Interestingly, in Geraldine's case, L'hermitte's sign gradually decreased over the years.

Another patient, Harriet, a 46-year-old woman with confirmed spinal cord compression at C5,6, described her symptoms as:

'an unbearable buzzing sensation down the neck and back.'

She went on to describe this sensation as:

'much more of a problem than the pain. ... The sensation is just like an intense electric shock.'

Clinicians should be alert to these types of descriptions as well as to the more classic orthopaedic version.

Discussion

People with MS often present early in the disease process with very subtle signs. One of those signs appears to be back pain. Interestingly, as in Geraldine's case, although other problems manifest themselves it is often the back pain which appears to be the most problematic symptom leading to an orthopaedic referral.

From a geographical perspective, clinicians should note that the prevalence of MS appears to be directly proportional to the distance of the location of the sufferer from the equator, i.e. the further north or south from the equator, the greater the prevalence of the condition. This will influence the conditional probability of whether the patient consulting with back pain may also be suffering from MS.

- Latitudes 50–65° north – prevalence 60–100/100 000
- Latitudes <30° north – prevalence 10/100 000
- At the equator – rare

(Kumar & Clark 2005)

CASE 2: FERGUS

In April 2006, Fergus, a 25-year-old manual worker, got out of his car at work and fell awkwardly down a deep hole dug in the ground, the left leg going down the hole up to thigh level, the right leg being outside the hole. He sustained a direct injury to the left buttock and pelvis and felt pain immediately. He struggled to sit and walk and so was immediately taken to the local A&E. At A&E, analgesia was administered and advice was given but no X-ray was done. Symptoms continued over the subsequent weeks with some paraesthesia in the upper left thigh but no radicular pain below the knee. However, Fergus reported that he had been impotent since the accident.

 What are you thinking now?

Consequently, Fergus was seen on an urgent basis on receipt of the referral. He described constant pain in the left lumbar spine and left hemi-pelvis along with some increased pain in the right testicle. Not only had he been unable to obtain a full erection but he also complained of saddle numbness. He described one possible episode of retention but this was not ongoing. A cough and sneeze increased low back pain and sacral pain. He was very stiff first thing in the morning and struggled to get going. His sleep was disturbed between four and six times a night when he tried to roll over or change positions. Symptoms were aggravated by sitting, walking, bending and crouching. Symptoms were eased to some degree by ice on the sacrum and very gentle massage. There was no past medical history of note; he was attempting to control his pain with a combination of non-steroidal anti-inflammatory drugs (NSAIDs) and analgesics.

On examination, Fergus walked with an antalgic gait and stood with the left knee flexed. Active movement testing revealed that all lumbar movements were restricted and painful; the pain was isolated to the left sacrum and hemi-pelvis. Throughout the examination it was obvious he had difficulty moving around, particularly standing to sitting and sitting to lying. Hip flexion bilaterally was restricted to 90°, increasing sacral pain. Straight leg raise bilaterally was restricted to 60°, increasing sacral pain once more. Apart from the impotence there were no other neurological deficits. Direct pressure on the sacrum and lateral pressure over the sacro-iliac joint increased his acute pain locally. He had some sensation loss in the perineum and the upper inner thigh but nothing else of note.

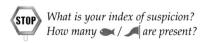

What is your index of suspicion?
How many 🐟 / 🐟 are present?

What are your diagnostic alternatives?
What will you do next with this patient?

There was no strong evidence of cauda equina syndrome (CES). However, the clinician felt that there was a possibility Fergus had a sacral fracture or fracture around the pelvic region and so organized an urgent X-ray. If the X-ray was negative, investigations would progress to a computed tomography (CT) or bone scan. The X-ray was negative and so an urgent CT scan was arranged. Similarly, this was also negative. However, during this short period, Fergus continued to suffer from severe low back and left leg pain associated with erectile dysfunction. Medical advice was sought and a stronger combination of medication was prescribed. This pain management strategy attempted to facilitate an early paced exercise approach, to improve his mobility. Physiotherapy was prescribed to assist with this care package.

One month later at his review appointment, there was actually some improvement; he was generally moving better and the erectile dysfunction was possibly now reversing. He was attempting to be more active and going for a daily walk.

At his next review appointment, three months after the injury, however, the presentation was more concerning for a different reason. He appeared to be spiralling into a chronic disability situation because of his condition. He appeared low in mood; he described pain from his lumber spine up to his cervical spine. His sleep pattern was disturbed and he was only sleeping for four hours at a time and lying on the settee during the day. His only exercise was walking the children to school but generally he seemed very lethargic and low. He did describe a need to get back to work as soon as possible due to financial pressures but felt that he would be unable to, due to the discomfort in his spine. The Roland and Morris Disability Questionnaire (R&MDQ) (Roland & Morris 1983) and the Linton and Halden initial back pain questionnaire (Linton & Halden 1998) were completed and identified that Fergus was now significantly disabled with his pain and was kinesophobic and markedly pessimistic about his future.

On examination there was evidence of a pain system dysfunction with no true neurological deficit. He described episodes of impotence but no disturbance of bladder or bowel function. He still described marked pain and discomfort in the genital region. Despite all efforts to control the pain and assist Fergus with his mobility, four months after his injury, he was referred to a pain management programme.

Discussion

A flag system highlighting risk factors has been developed to alert clinicians that there may be a poor outcome in some patients with low back pain for reasons other than biomedical. According to Robson (2007), within physiotherapy practice:

'The incorporation of the coloured flags concept over the last ten years or so has become an essential adjunct to their traditional hands-on skills.'

The following flag system highlights these psychosocial indicators (Main 2004):

- Yellow Flags – psychological and behavioural factors
- Blue Flags – perceptions of work and working conditions:
  - High demand and low control
  - Time pressure/monotonous work
  - Lack of job satisfaction
  - Low social support from colleagues
  - High perceived workload
- Black Flags – sickness management policy and socioeconomic policy:
  - Specific job characteristics
  - Management style
  - Social climate
- Orange Flags – psychiatric factors:
  - Major personality disorder
  - Illicit drug use
  - Forensic issues
  - Major communication problems
  - Active psychiatric disorder

It is interesting to consider the complex psychosocial and biomedical picture that emerges in the case of Fergus. He presents with a combination of Red, Yellow, Blue and Black Flags. In the case of Fergus, the initial clinical presentation was with what appeared to be a host of clear Red Flags. Through a logical process of appropriate investigations, the Red Flags proved to be negative. With time the clinical picture steadily metamorphosized into one of unmistakable psychosocial risk factors rather than serious pathology indictors.

However, we would like to re-emphasize that it is essential to conduct diagnostic triage in the first instance, identifying any Red Flags and instigating appropriate further investigation or management/ onward referral as soon as possible. It is also important to remember that Red Flags can emerge at any time in the disease process and so continuous assessment of the patient's condition is essential. Similarly, those patients who have presented for many years with Yellow Flags are not immune to serious spinal pathology and can at some stage develop a biomedical problem, with Red Flags beginning to subtly emerge under cover of a chronic disability and/or maladaptive illness behaviour. It is always vitally important to establish from the patient's subjective history:

'Is this pain different from your usual pain?'

ALCOHOLISM

Patients with alcoholism can sometimes present a confusing clinical picture (Johnston 1999). There is no specific blood test for detecting alcoholism. The most common tests for alcoholism are liver function tests; these primarily assess liver injury (alcoholic hepatitis) rather than liver function. It should be noted that liver function tests are not specific and may indicate problems arising outside the liver such as bone disease reflected in elevated alkaline phosphatase levels. Derek's case in

Chapter 6 provides a good example of this as his cirrhosis had developed as a consequence of a genetic predisposition, rather than alcoholism.

Two of the key markers of hepatic injury are aspartate aminotransferase (AST) and alanine aminotransferase (ALT) (Johnston 1999). ALT is the most sensitive marker for liver cell damage as it is normally only found in the liver (Jensen & Freese 2006). Interpretation of tests demonstrating raised levels for these two enzymes needs to be performed cautiously as neither follows a normal bell-shaped distribution in healthy populations; the distributions are positively skewed with a long tail to the right (see Chapter 8). ALT distributions in particular are skewed in this direction in males and non-white races so that more values fall at or above the upper defined limits of normal (Johnston 1999).

In patients with alcoholic hepatitis the serum AST level is almost never greater than 500 U/L and the serum ALT value is almost never greater than 300 U/L. In addition, in alcoholic hepatitis, the ratio of AST to ALT is greater than 1 and is usually greater than 2, and the higher this ratio the greater the likelihood that alcohol is contributing to the abnormal test result (Johnston 1999). Following cell death, enzymes are released; these provide clues as to the type of cell affected, e.g. ALT is specific for the liver.

Signs and symptoms of alcoholism (Essortment 2006; Johnston 1999) are:

- Unexplained mood swings, depression and irritability
- Abdominal pain

- Fever
- Weakness and numbness in the limbs
- Loss of interest in social activities
- Neglect of physical appearance
- Eating disorders and poor diet leading to weight loss

Some of these symptoms also appear as Red Flags for serious spinal pathology and many of these are found in the prodromal phase of serious pathology. In cases of alcoholism, clinicians need to be careful in interpreting the whole clinical picture as these symptoms can easily be misinterpreted presenting as Red Herrings. Apart from raised AST and ALT levels, prolonged heavy alcohol consumption can lead to the other abnormalities (Wikipedia 2006):

- Raised mean corpuscular volume (MCV) (macrocytosis)
- Elevated gamma-glutamyl transpeptidase (GGT)

Macrocytosis is the enlargement of red blood cells but with a near-constant haemoglobin concentration. Macrocytosis is usually defined as having MCV levels in excess of 100 femtolitres. GGT is a liver enzyme which, when raised, may indicate hepatic abnormality such as liver tumour. Levels can also be raised in congestive cardiac failure and in alcoholism (Wikipedia 2006).

THYROID FUNCTION DISORDERS

Hypothyroidism may mimic many rheumatic diseases (Waltuck 2001). The incidence of musculoskeletal symptoms in hypothyroidism has been reported to be as high as 30–80% (Khaleeli et al 1983). However, many patients will be unaware that they have a thyroid condition or that their thyroid condition is causing their musculoskeletal symptoms. For these reasons abnormalities of the thyroid should be considered when assessing a patient with musculoskeletal problems (Waltuck 2001).

Signs and symptoms of hypothyroidism (Brady 2000; Waltuck 2001) are:

- Fatigue/lethargy
- Cold intolerance
- Swelling of hands, feet and face
- Chronic infections
- Weakness
- Cramp
- Arthralgia with joint effusion
- Paraesthesia
- Carpal tunnel syndrome (10% incidence of hypothyroidism in patients with carpal tunnel syndrome)
- Constipation
- Morning stiffness

Many of the musculoskeletal symptoms are thought to occur as a result of oedema formation in the joints and soft tissues (Brady 2000). Hypothyroidism is relatively common in middle-aged women and can manifest itself in a very similar way to fibromyalgia. However, in contrast to patients with fibromyalgia, patients with hypothyroidism rarely complain of sleep disturbance, irritable bowels, headaches and palpitations.

A homeostatic loop between the thyroid and pituitary glands is maintained by the production of thyroxine (T4) from the thyroid gland and thyroid stimulating hormone (TSH) from the pituitary gland. Interestingly, a high TSH level actually indicates a primary problem in the thyroid gland as the pituitary gland will produce excess quantities of TSH in an attempt to stimulate the thyroid gland into producing more T4. T4 circulates in the blood in two forms, bound to protein or free (FT4). Combining the results of TSH and FT4 testing gives an accurate picture of how the thyroid gland is functioning. Elevated TSH and low FT4 indicate primary hypothyroidism due to disease in the thyroid gland. Low TSH and low FT4 indicate hypothyroidism due to a pituitary problem (American Thyroid Association 2005).

DIABETES MELLITUS

Diabetes mellitus (DM) is a multi-system disease characterized by persistent hyperglycaemia. Type 1 DM is relatively rare and usually occurs in children and young adults up to the early 40s. Type 2 DM is much more common, occurring in approximately 90% of cases, and typically in older obese individuals. Both types appear to have some genetic disposition so information regarding family history may be an important area to explore during the subjective examination (Wyatt & Ferrance 2006).

Musculoskeletal effects of DM are listed below with the percentage of diabetic patients presenting with the condition in parenthesis where available (Wyatt & Ferrance 2006):

- Muscle cramp
- Muscle infarction
- Loss of deep tendon reflexes
- Peripheral neuropathy
- Complex regional pain syndrome (CRPS)
- Stiff hands syndrome (50% in type 1 DM)
- Neuropathic joints (1%)
- Carpal tunnel syndrome (30%)
- Frozen shoulder (20%)
- Tenosynovitis
- Diffuse idiopathic skeletal hyperostosis (DISH) (26%)
- Ossification of the posterior longitudinal ligament (OPLL)
- Dupuytren's contracture (>33%)

The prevalence of many of these conditions increases with the duration of diabetes.

A blood glucose test measures the amount of glucose in the blood; it can be used to detect both hyperglycaemia and hypoglycaemia and helps to diagnose diabetes (Lab Tests Online 2005; Table 7.1). Clinicians should be aware that many different versions of the test exist and they should check locally to confirm which method is preferred in their area.

Table 7.1 Differential diagnosis of altered glucose levels (Lab Tests Online 2005)

Hyperglycaemia	Hypoglycaemia
Acromegaly	Adrenal insufficiency
Acute stress response to trauma (heart attack, stroke)	Alcoholism
Chronic renal failure	Drugs
Cushing syndrome	Hepatic disease
Drugs	Hypopituitarism
Hyperthyroidism	Hypothyroidism
Pancreatitis and pancreatic cancer	Insulin overdose
	Insulinomas
	Starvation

DISCUSSION

We first introduced the term Red Herrings in the paper *Margaret: a tragic case of spinal Red Flags and Red Herrings* (Greenhalgh & Selfe 2004). We considered the term to be broad and to encompass any misleading biomedical or psychosocial factors that could deflect the course of accurate clinical reasoning. We followed up this by presenting the following list of Red Herrings (Greenhalgh & Selfe 2006):

- Misattribution by:
  - Patient
  - Referring doctor or allied health professional
  - Treating physiotherapist

- Inappropriate overt illness behaviour
- Other conditions which complicate the clinical scenario but which do not impact on the management of the patient
- Biomedical masqueraders

One of the important areas we would like to focus on here is how the availability of an increasing battery of diagnostic tests can lead to misattribution by health professionals. There are two issues: first, the ordering of the correct test appropriate to the patient's condition, and second, interpretation of the test results when they become available.

Clinicians may derive false reassurance from the normal results of tests that do not actually address the appropriate clinical question (Lewis 2004). Therefore when ordering a test it is vital that a robust clinical reasoning process has led to a conclusion of the greatest belief, which supports the decision to order a specific test or group of tests rather than the test/s forming part of a clinical 'fishing expedition' in the hope of finding something. It is important to remember that, statistically, the more tests you order the more likely you will eventually find an incidental abnormal result (Deyo & Hope 2005) or that a false-positive result will be returned.

Clinical interpretation of a patient's tests results in isolation from the subjective, and objective examination is also potentially very hazardous (Lewis 2004). Edith's case in Chapter 5 provides a very good example of this, where test results were interpreted by a clinician who had never seen the patient. Eminent authorities such as Deyo & Hope (2005) state that the:

'Interpretation of test results is rarely straightforward'.

Incidental abnormalities can also be over-interpreted with respect to their clinical importance. It is interesting to note that back surgery rates are highest where MRI rates are highest (Deyo & Hope 2005). MRI scans reveal tiny abnormalities which may simply represent normal human variation that would have once gone unnoticed. Many of these abnormalities are trivial, harmless and clinically irrelevant which has led to the coining of the interesting term 'incidentalomas' (Deyo & Hope 2005).

In Chapter 2 we briefly discussed the methodological concepts associated with the sensitivity and specificity of tests. It is worth revisiting these concepts here, as associated with most tests there will be false positives, i.e. the test result will be positive despite the patient not having the condition under investigation, and false negatives, i.e. the test result will be negative despite the patient actually having the condition being tested for. Deyo & Hope (2005) caution against placing too much emphasis on one test result. In practice, it is important that the results of different tests are 'triangulated' with clinical impressions in order to increase confidence that the patient does or does not have the condition of interest.

Clinicians have to tread a fine line between ordering enough tests to confirm a particular diagnosis and not ordering too many that will lead to an increased chance of finding a false-positive result. We will go on to discuss issues around ordering and interpreting tests in the next chapter.

References

American Thyroid Association 2005 Thyroid function tests. Online. Available: www.thyroid.org (accessed 6 July 2006)

Brady D 2000 Functional thyroid disorders. Dynamic Chiropractic 18: 1–7

Deyo R A, Hope D L 2005 Hope or hype. AMACOM, New York

Essortment 2006 Signs and symptoms of alcoholism. Online. Available: http://www.essortment.com (accessed 5 July 2006)

Greenhalgh S, Selfe J 2004 Margaret: a tragic case of spinal Red Flags and Red Herrings. Physiotherapy 90: 73–76

Greenhalgh S, Selfe J 2006 Red Flags: a guide to identifying serious pathology of the spine, 1st edn. Churchill Livingstone, Elsevier, Edinburgh

Jensen J E, Freese D 2006 Liver function tests. Online. Available: www.gastromed.com/lft.html (accessed 27 June 2006)

Johnston D E 1999 Special considerations in interpreting liver function tests. American Family Physician 59: 1–11

Khaleeli A A, Griffith D H, Edwards R H T 1983 The clinical presentation of hypothyroid myopathy and its relationship to abnormalities in structure and function of skeletal muscle. Clinical Endocrinology 19: 365–376

Kumar P, Clark M 2005 Clinical medicine, 6th edn. W B Saunders, Edinburgh

Lab Tests Online 2005 Online. Available: www.labtestsonline.org (accessed 6 July 2006)

Lewis S L 2004 An approach to neurologic symptoms. In: Weiner W J, Goetz C G (eds) Neurology for the non-neurologist, 5th edn. Lippincott Williams & Wilkins, Philadelphia

Linton S J, Halden K 1998 Can we screen for problematic back pain? A screening questionnaire for predicting outcome in acute and subacute back pain. Clinical Journal of Pain 14: 200–215

Main C 2004 Psychosocial factors: their identification and management in consultation with physiotherapists. McKenzie Institute Journal Denmark 14: 11–14

Robson S 2007 Editorial. Physiotherapy Pain Association Newsletter. December

Roland M, Morris R W 1983 A study of the natural history of back pain. Part 1: development of a reliable and sensitive measure of disability in low back pain. Spine 8: 141–144

Waltuck J 2001 Musculoskeletal manifestations of thyroid disease. Bulletin on the Rheumatic Diseases 49: 1–3

Wikipedia 2006 Online. Available: http://en.wikipedia.org (accessed 5 July 2006)

Wyatt L H, Ferrance R J 2006 The musculoskeletal effects of diabetes mellitus. Journal of the Canadian Chiropractic Association 50: 43–50

Chapter 8

Investigations in Serious Pathology of the Spine

Andrew Maskell, Sue Greenhalgh,
James Selfe

In the field of musculoskeletal medicine, when suspecting the possibility of serious pathology of the spine, common questions are generated by clinicians within the clinical reasoning process during the search for a definitive diagnosis, such as:

- Where do I start?
- What blood test should I do?
- This blood result is abnormal but is it significant?
- Should I take an X-ray of the spine?
- Should I order a magnetic resonance (MR) scan?
- Does the patient need a bone scan?
- Does my patient need a combination of investigations?
- If so – which combination would be appropriate?

The correct starting point should always be a detailed history and a thorough examination, and the ordering of investigation results must be based on those findings. Furthermore, interpretation of investigation results should always be in the clinical context of the patient's condition and past history; a failure to do this runs the risk of identifying Red Herrings leading to inappropriate treatment pathways. For example, results of blood tests can be chronically abnormal and many abnormalities reported on MR scans are either age-related degenerative phenomena irrelevant to the patient's immediate condition or incidental findings of no clinical significance. Careful interpretation of results in the immediate clinical context is therefore essential.

This chapter will discuss common blood pathology and radiology investigations used to assist the musculoskeletal clinician in reaching a diagnosis or differential diagnosis and thus ensure that the patient is referred to the correct service and the most appropriate treatment gets underway without delay, i.e.

'Right person, right place, right time'.

SHOULD I ORDER ANY INVESTIGATIONS AT ALL?

If serious pathology is suspected, appropriate further investigations should be considered (Bogduk & McGuirk 2002). However, unnecessary investigations not only waste valuable time and resources but can also cause unnecessary anxiety and distress for the patient, family and friends (Levack et al 2002). If the therapist is in any doubt about whether to order a test or if there is any uncertainty in the interpretation of the test result, they should always discuss this with the appropriate medical, pathology or radiology staff. Prior to ordering investigations, the clinician must consider (Asher 1954):

- Why do I order these tests?
- What am I going to look for in the result?
- If I find it, will it affect my diagnosis?
- How will this affect my management of the case?
- Will this ultimately benefit the patient?

Another way of looking at this is to consider three important premises before ordering a test:

- Aim to do investigations that prove what you already suspect and/or know
- Be willing and able to interpret and act on the results
- Be prepared to deal with the unexpected

The worst thing to do is to arrange investigations just because one doesn't know what to do next. In this situation, it is almost inevitable that the results will turn up more questions than answers! It is always better to seek another opinion than waste time on unnecessary and/or inappropriate investigations.

ASSESSING RISK

Bogduk & McGuirk (2002) suggest that any patient with a past history of cancer should be considered 'high risk' and further investigations considered. An erythrocyte sedimentation rate (ESR) and appropriate imaging are recommended. The method of imaging depends on the patient and nature of the suspected pathology.

Patients of 50 years or more who are not responding to conservative management, with unexplained weight loss and systemically unwell are considered as 'intermediate risk'. These cases warrant an ESR. If the ESR is raised (Bogduk & McGuirk suggest an ESR of more than 20 mm/h), further imaging is advised. Patients younger than 50 years of age with no systemic illness, history of cancer or weight loss, and who make steady improvements with simple conservative measures are considered 'low risk'. No investigations are suggested in these cases.

BLOOD PATHOLOGY

Common blood pathology tests are divided into:

- Haematology
- Biochemistry
- Immunology

For the purposes of this book, we will give guidance on some relevant blood tests considered within the field of musculoskeletal medicine when a diagnosis of serious pathology of the spine is suspected, with a full blood count, ESR, basic biochemical tests, prostate-specific antigen (PSA) and protein electrophoresis being the most useful (Kumar & Clark 2005).

Most blood test results are now generated by automated machines and are therefore inexpensive and rapidly available. In urgent cases, common blood results can be obtained within minutes of the sample being obtained. Although most samples are processed in hospital laboratory departments, the simplification of analytical equipment now means that many simple tests can be processed on portable equipment away from a central laboratory.

WHAT IS NORMAL?

The range of results for a given blood test that can be considered 'normal' is based on a statistical analysis of the distribution of results in healthy individuals. In a conventional normal distribution, most of the values are clustered around the mean value with fewer results lying further away. The distribution of values is also symmetrical, giving the classical 'bell shape' to the curve when they are plotted graphically (Fig. 8.1).

By statistical analysis, it can be demonstrated that about 95% of results lie within 2 standard deviations (SD) of the mean value and this is referred to as the 'normal range'. It is often referred to as the 95% confidence interval and indicates the likelihood of the value outside the normal range not being due to chance.

For pathology results, the normal range is often indicated on result forms as a range of values in brackets, sometimes supplemented with an 'H' (high) or 'L' (low) if the result is above or below this range, respectively. If a value lies outside this normal range then it is usually assumed to be abnormal, although one should remember that statistically 5% of values will still lie outside this range in a population of healthy individuals.

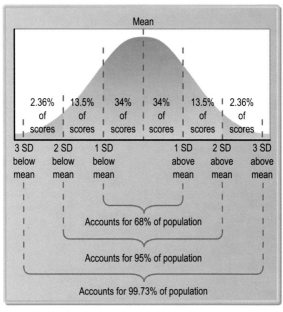

Fig. 8.1 A typical normal distribution showing how values are distributed symmetrically around the mean (µ) with 95% of the values lying within 2 SD (±2 SD) of the mean (Hicks 2009).

WHEN IS AN ABNORMAL RESULT SIGNIFICANT?

Perhaps the best way to understand the significance of an abnormal result is to get used to looking at lots of normal results obtained in situations where serious pathology is considered unlikely. It will become apparent that the occasional abnormal result occurs in these situations and confidence can be gained in understanding that these minor variations can occur in healthy individuals and when other, less serious conditions are being assessed. It will then become more evident when abnormal results should be taken as an indication of a potentially serious disorder. Usually, individual results that are just outside the normal range can be considered acceptable, but when several results are outside the normal range or an individual result is some way beyond the normal range, it more likely indicates a potentially serious problem.

It is useful to understand normal homeostatic processes and to look at the range of normal values in this context. For example, the normal plasma concentration of sodium is much higher than potassium, typical mean values being 140 mmol/L and 4.0 mmol/L, respectively. Plasma potassium levels are also much more tightly controlled than sodium levels with smaller variations being associated with ill health. Consequently, the normal range of sodium levels (typically 135–145 mmol/L) is much wider than potassium levels (3.5–4.5 mmol/L). It therefore follows that a sodium level of 146 mmol/L (just 1 mmol/L above the normal range) is unlikely to be all that remarkable whereas a potassium level that is 1 mmol/L above the normal range at 5.5 mmol/L certainly would be. More critical is the plasma calcium level which is even more tightly controlled (normal range 2.15–2.62 mmol/L) where a rise of 1 mmol/L above the normal range to 3.62 mmol/L could not only indicate a need for emergency treatment but potentially be even fatal.

SKEWED DISTRIBUTIONS

Things can get a little more complicated when the distribution of 'normal' values is skewed one way or the other. In this situation, the greater mass of values lies towards one side of the distribution curve, as demonstrated in Figure 8.2.

A good example of this is the ESR, where the value is rarely below 2–3 mm/h, the mean value is typically 5 mm/h, and results up to 20 mm/h can be considered perfectly acceptable in many healthy individuals. This represents a 'positive skew'. Furthermore, the degree of 'skewness', indicated by the length of the longer tail,

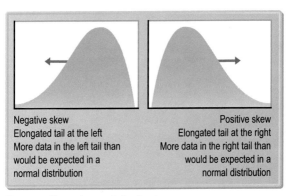

Negative skew
Elongated tail at the left
More data in the left tail than
would be expected in a
normal distribution

Positive skew
Elongated tail at the right
More data in the right tail than
would be expected in a
normal distribution

Fig. 8.2 Skewed normal distributions.

can vary with age, with older patients typically having a higher ESR. In this situation, it can be much more difficult to decide whether a raised ESR is significant or not. Even so, an ESR of 40 mm/h or more should definitely raise concern.

WATCH THE TREND

Sometimes, the best way to asses whether an abnormal result is significant or not is to repeat the test after an interval. If the repeat result is worse than before then it makes it more likely that the result indicates significant problems. If the repeat result has returned towards normal then it is less likely to be significant. It is also useful to obtain results for a test done previous to presentation as these can sometimes identify results that are chronically abnormal. For example, the ESR can be chronically elevated after a previous systemic illness. An ESR of 40 mm/h is much less worrying if it is known that it has been chronically elevated at this level for several years. If the ESR was only 5 mm/h a year ago then it would make a current ESR of 40 mm/h of far greater concern, even more so if it had risen to 60 mm/h after another short interval.

VARIATION OF NORMAL RANGES

Reference ranges used for blood cell counts originate from clinical trials in the early 1960s and vary little from site to site. However, reference ranges for biochemistry results quoted in textbooks and journal papers should be considered for guidance only, as methods of analysis can vary significantly from one laboratory to another. In addition, as methodology changes in line with the introduction of new techniques, the ranges become outdated and are therefore subject to constant review. It should also be remembered that ranges may be affected by issues such as:

- Age
- Gender
- Ethnic group
- Pregnancy
- Time of sampling
- Storage and transport

Detailed information or advice on interpretation of results is always available from the local laboratory staff (Squire 2003).

HAEMATOLOGY

FULL BLOOD COUNT

Obtaining a full blood count (FBC) gives information about the numbers and types of cell in blood. Cells that circulate in the blood stream are divided into three main types:

- Red blood cells (erythrocytes)
- White blood cells (leucocytes)
- Platelets (thrombocytes)

High or low cell counts outside the normal ranges can indicate the presence of many diseases, hence blood counts are among the most commonly performed blood tests. An FBC provides non-specific information and it does not identify the particular cause or site of pathology. It does, however, provide helpful screening information when a problem is suspected.

Anaemia (RBC, MCHC and MCV)

Anaemia is the lack of haemoglobin carrying capacity in the blood, which might be due to a reduction in the red blood cell (RBC) count, a drop in the concentration of haemoglobin within the red blood cells (mean cell hemoglobin concentration (MCHC)), a change in red blood cell size (mean corpuscular volume (MCV)) or a combination of these.

There are many causes of anaemia (McGhee 2005). Mild anaemia frequently occurs in elderly individuals due to the effects of ageing and chronic illness, and so the whole clinical presentation must be considered and appropriate clinical reasoning applied if anaemia is found (McGhee 2005). Anaemia can occur in anyone who is unwell, particularly when suffering from malignancy or infection.

The pathological causes of anaemia can be complex. In cases of myeloma, for example, the increased numbers of abnormal plasma cells reduces the bone marrow's capacity to make normal red blood cells, causing anaemia (Net Doctor 2008). The MCV can rise or fall in anaemia. If the MCV is below the normal range (microcytic anaemia), this usually indicates some form of iron deficiency problem, most commonly due to poor dietary intake or occult blood loss due to internal bleeding. This picture is frequently found in serious pathology scenarios.

A raised MCV (macrocytic anaemia) often relates to a deficiency of vitamin B_{12} or folic acid, essential for DNA synthesis and cell replication, and is more likely to be dietary or metabolic in origin. However, macrocytosis can also occur as a result of cell toxicity from certain types of chemotherapy and drug treatment. It is also commonly associated with excess alcohol consumption due to bone marrow toxicity, when the MCV can frequently rise above 100 fL. It is useful to look at the aspartate transaminase (AST) or gamma-glutamyl transpeptidase (GGT or gamma-GT) levels as these will also tend to rise in chronic alcohol consumption.

WHITE BLOOD CELL COUNT

The white blood cell (WBC) count represents the total number of WBCs in the whole blood sample and can rise or fall in a number of scenarios. In cases of serious pathology, it is more common to find the WBC count rising (leucocytosis) in response to some form of 'inflammatory' process. This most commonly indicates a bacterial infection but can occur in almost any form of acute illness and is frequently seen in cases of malignancy.

In more serious cases, the WBC count can fall (leucopenia) as the consumption of WBCs outstrips the bone marrow's ability to produce them. This can be seen in the early stages of acute septicaemia, when the WBCs are migrating from the blood stream at a high rate to combat infection before the bone marrow has had time to respond to the increased demand, or where the bone marrow production has been suppressed (myelo-suppression), frequently due to malignant bone marrow infiltration or the effects of drug treatment.

In order to understand these processes better it is useful to look at the proportions of the different types of WBCs given in a differential count. This can be reported as absolute numbers of the different types of WBCs, the proportions of the different cell types as a percentage of the total, or both. A rise in the neutrophil count is usually associated with more acute inflammatory responses such as bacterial infections and advancing malignancy. A rise in the lymphocyte count is more commonly associated with chronic disorders and is frequently seen in tuberculosis for example.

If the blood cell count is markedly abnormal, the laboratory will often report on the appearances of a blood smear. This can give some indication as to the visible characteristics of the blood cells. In cases where production of new cells is high, the blood cells will often take on a more immature form, the cells being larger and with more densely packed nuclei, often referred to as a 'left shift'.

ERYTHROCYTE SEDIMENTATION RATE

If normal blood is left to stand in a tube, the RBCs will gradually fall towards the bottom of the sample under the influence of gravity. This effect can be measured by the erythrocyte sedimentation rate (ESR), in which the distance the cells fall is measured over a fixed time interval. In most laboratory tests, a sample of whole blood is drawn up into a capillary tube that is then sealed and left to stand vertically in a standardized environment for one hour. A technician then measures how far the RBCs have fallen and the result is given in mm/h. From this it can be understood that this test is both labour intensive and time consuming. An ESR specimen also needs careful storage and transport and is best stored in a vertical position and processed within two hours of collection (McGhee 2005). For these reasons, many laboratories are moving to replace ESR measurements with other related, automated tests such as plasma viscosity (PV). However, ESR is still considered to be a good screening test for suspected serious pathology in the spine.

The ESR varies greatly in different physiologies and pathological conditions. It is influenced by age, gender and any concurrent anaemia.

A useful rule of thumb is that a patient's ESR should be less than their age minus 20, divided by two;

$$(Age - 20)/2 = acceptable ESR$$

e.g. in the case of a 66-year-old, an acceptable ESR would be:

$$(66 - 20)/2 = 23 \text{ mm/h}$$

Elevated plasma proteins also increase the rate at which the RBCs settle. An ESR is a useful indicator of serious pathology but is not diagnostic, and to establish its true significance a series of ESR measurements should be taken over a period of time. This could be weeks, or even months, but in cases of more systemic illness, this may be days. It is important to remember that the rise and, especially, fall of the ESR often lags behind the clinical condition by sometimes weeks or even months. The ESR can also remain chronically elevated long after a condition has resolved. Any single result over 50 mm/h is generally immediately indicative of a serious disease process but a series of results might still be considered and a repeat ESR is generally suggested after two weeks, or earlier if the patient's condition is deteriorating. A high ESR can occur in many conditions, but with respect to the spine these include malignancy (especially malignant myeloma, where an ESR above 100 is almost diagnostic), acute bacterial infection (including tuberculosis), auto-immune disease and following trauma (McGhee 2005).

However, on occasions a moderately elevated result (20–50 mm/h) might raise false suspicion. If the ESR is slightly raised, always aim to check a series of results (but only if time permits) and always remember to compare with any results available from previous tests to establish if there is an increasing trend.

BIOCHEMISTRY

C-REACTIVE PROTEIN

CRP is an acute phase protein, largely produced in the liver, and released in inflammatory processes. It is, therefore, raised in infections but, importantly, not raised in all cases of malignancy; thus in some cases of malignancy the CRP can be normal (McGhee 2005). A raised CRP also appears during acute tissue necrosis within 24–48 hours.

The normal range is below 5 mg/L. If levels are around 50 mg/L or above, the underlying condition is often serious. The CRP changes much more rapidly than the ESR and does not suffer from the same lag in response time. Serial CRP measurements can be particularly helpful in monitoring cases of infection or inflammatory disease and their response to treatment. This time frame can be condition specific and can range from days to weeks or months in the case of more chronic conditions such as rheumatoid arthritis.

CALCIUM METABOLISM

Calcium is the most common mineral in the human body, there being approximately 1500 g of calcium in the adult body. Most of this calcium is used in the structure of bone and bone forms a substantial calcium store. However, calcium also plays an important role in the following processes (McArdle et al 1991):

- Muscle contraction
- Transmission of nerve impulses
- Enzyme reactions
- Blood clotting
- Fluid transport across cell membranes

The blood plasma calcium level is closely regulated within a small range by the body. Calcium is carried in the blood in several forms but the most important are free ionic calcium and that bound to albumin. The plasma calcium level therefore varies with the level of albumin. The total calcium (also referred to as the corrected calcium) can be calculated if the albumin level is known:

$$\text{Total calcium} = \text{Measured calcium} + (0.02 \times (40 - \text{albumin level}))$$

Calcium metabolism is largely regulated by the parathyroid glands and kidneys and involves three hormones:

- Vitamin D, produced in a complex metabolic process involving the skin, liver and kidney
- Parathyroid hormone (PTH), produced by the parathyroid glands
- Calcitonin, produced in the parafollicular C-cells in the thyroid

The inter-relationships between these three hormones are complex but, in simple terms, vitamin D is required for the absorption of calcium and its integration into bone stores, PTH raises calcium levels in the blood, and calcitonin lowers the blood calcium level.

Total calcium of more than 2.6 mmol/L indicates hypercalcaemia. Hypercalcaemia is a potentially serious condition. The calcium level can rise slowly with little effect on the patient's well-being but sometimes it can rise rapidly causing acute collapse. A calcium level above 3 mmol/L often requires emergency treatment with correction of fluid balance, steroids and sometimes calcitonin therapy. The symptoms of hypercalcaemia are variable and are associated more with the rate of change of calcium level rather than absolute level of calcium (Binns & Gurney 1998).

Symptoms of hypercalcaemia, often summarized as

'bone, stones, moans and abdominal groans'

include (Kochhar & Marshall 2003; Oken 2002):

- Pain
- Weakness
- Constipation
- Depression
- Tiredness/lethargy
- Nausea/vomiting
- Thirst
- Poor appetite
- Formation of renal stones

One of the most common reasons for hypercalcaemia is malignancy. Up to 30% of all cancer patients will develop hypercalcaemia (Medline Plus 2005) and 50% of all patients diagnosed with hypercalcaemia will have a malignant disease (Binns & Gurney 1998). The majority of patients with severe hypercalcaemia will have metastases identifiable on X-rays or isotope bone scans (Souhami & Tobias 1995). Hypercalcaemia does not result from bone destruction by metastases per se but due to hormonal release by tumours which activate osteoclasts and interfere with kidney regulation. Patients with hypercalcaemia are at increased risk of cardiac arrest (Oken 2002).

Malignancies particularly associated with hypercalcaemia include (Cancer Research UK 2006; Medline Plus 2005; Oken 2002):

- Multiple myeloma (33% of myeloma patients will develop hypercalcaemia)
- Breast tumours
- Squamous cell lung tumours
- Renal cell tumours

PROSTATE-SPECIFIC ANTIGEN

PSA is a protein produced by the prostate and released in very small amounts into the blood stream. When prostate cancer develops, more PSA is released, until it reaches a level where it can be detected easily in the blood. The range for PSA levels are as follows:

- Under 4 µg/mL – usually considered normal
- Between 4 µg/mL to 10 µg/mL – usually considered intermediate
- Over 10 µg/mL – considered high

An elevated PSA that continues to rise is a strong indicator of prostatic malignancy, and the higher the level, the greater the likelihood of the tumour having metastasized (Prostate Cancer Research Foundation 2008).

IMMUNOLOGY

PROTEIN ELECTROPHORESIS

Within the field of musculoskeletal medicine, protein electrophoresis is commonly used to screen for myeloma (Kumar & Clark 2005). The screening tests for myeloma in routine practice should be both serum and urine electrophoresis. If these are both negative, myeloma is exceedingly unlikely.

While a high ESR of 60 mm/h or more is often suggestive of myeloma, a high ESR is not specific enough in isolation to make a diagnosis. This diagnosis requires two out of the following three to be positive:

- Serum and/or urine protein electrophoresis
- Radiographic skeletal survey
- Bone marrow aspirate examination

Characteristic appearances on a lateral skull X-ray ('pepper-pot skull') and a diagnostic bone marrow aspirate are specifically diagnostic for this condition.

Protein electrophoresis reveals the presence of the monoclonal antibodies produced in substantial quantities by these tumours.

Negative serum electrophoresis results are seen in light chain myeloma as the light chains are passed out in the urine. If only ESR and serum electrophoresis are requested then a patient with light chain myeloma could be missed.

In protein electrophoresis, the various proteins in serum, urine, or cerebrospinal fluid (CSF) can be separated. Along with albumin, other principal protein groups include (McGhee 2005):

- Albumin
- α_2-Globulins
- β-Globulins
- γ-Globulins

All γ-globulins are immunoglobulins of which IgG constitutes 75% of the total. To perform the test, the fluid to be analysed is dropped into wells cut into a thin layer of gel. An electrical current is passed through the gel. The distances proteins travel through the gel under the influence of the electrical charge depend on their individual size, shape and electrical charge. These separated proteins can be identified by the application of a dye to the gel plate that stains the proteins and reveals a characteristic pattern of bands. Each band represents a particular protein type and the width and/or density of the band is an indication of the quantity.

Multiple myeloma is associated with the uncontrolled proliferation of malignant plasma cells that are essentially all clones of the same cell line. These cells produce large quantities of the same immunoglobulin or immunoglobulin fragment, and it is this that produces the typical monoclonal band seen on protein electrophoresis (Lab Tests Online 2005). A discrete monoclonal γ-globulin band is almost immediately associated with myeloma. Other types of malignancy tend to cause a general rise in α_2-globulins (McGhee 2005).

Normally, the kidney retains plasma proteins in the blood so the abnormal monoclonal antibodies steadily accumulate. However, certain myeloma tumours (and occasionally other tumours) produce immunoglobulin fragments or 'paraproteins' known as Bence Jones proteins. These can be small enough to escape through the kidney and therefore appear in the urine rather than accumulating in the blood. Up to 15% of myeloma tumours produce these light chain immunoglobulin fragments and thus it is good practice to request urinary protein electrophoresis if myeloma is strongly suspected but the serum protein electrophoresis does not prove positive. Most laboratories can give a qualitative assessment of the presence of Bence Jones proteins on a single early morning sample of urine, when the urine is most concentrated, but a quantitative assessment usually requires a collection of urine over a 24-hour period (Wikipedia 2006).

RADIOLOGY

When considering which type of imaging to use, it is important to understand what the image can show, i.e. bone or soft tissue, how reliable is it, how specific is it and what are the potential hazards? Bogduk &

McGuirk (2002) suggest that diagnostic imaging be considered when one or more of the following items are present:

- History of cancer
- Unexplained weight loss
- Temperature >37.8°
- Risk factors of infection
- Neurological deficit
- Failure to improve
- Risk factors of fracture

Although radiology investigations are widely available, it should be remembered that there are risks associated with their use. Even plain radiographs, with their relatively low levels of irradiation, are not without hazard as the body tissues still absorb the radiation energy from the X-rays passed through them. A plain radiograph of the lumbar spine is estimated to deliver 40 times the radiation dose of a chest X-ray. Furthermore, the potential damage to the various structures exposed to an X-ray beam is not uniform. Put into context, an antero-posterior (AP) and lateral X-ray of the lumbar spine is said to deliver to the gonads a radiation dose equivalent to 1 daily chest X-ray for six years.

Acquiring and interpreting radiographic images is a highly skilled task and must always been done in the context of the clinical problem. Modern imaging techniques are highly sensitive and will detect many 'abnormalities' that are simply due to the effects of developmental variation or ageing. It is therefore essential to give the radiology team a clear explanation of the clinical problem and the questions needing to be answered on the referral form. Simply requesting an MR scan of the spine for 'back pain' is unacceptable and will usually result in the request for imaging being rejected. If there is any doubt as to the best imaging technique to use then the case should always be discussed first with a radiologist to avoid unnecessary delay.

PLAIN RADIOGRAPHS (X-RAYS)

Plain radiography involves passing an X-ray beam through the body and onto a flat film plate or digital detector. Body tissues of different density will absorb varying degrees of the X-ray beam thus casting a 'shadow' on the image. Hard tissue, such as bone, absorbs the greatest quantity of the X-ray beam and air-filled spaces, such as the lungs, the least. Traditionally, the image is processed and displayed in a negative sense such that the densest tissues, such as bone, show as white, or radio-dense, areas and the least dense tissues show as dark, or radiolucent, areas. The image generated is a two-dimensional representation of a three-dimensional structure and thus different structures can end up being superimposed on each other. In order to resolve this it is common practice to take radiographs in pairs at right angles (for example antero-posterior and lateral) to allow three-dimensional structures and their relationships to one another to be shown more clearly.

Plain radiography is probably the least helpful of the radiological modalities for identifying serious pathology of the spine. It is well recognized that up to 50% of a vertebral body needs to be destroyed before the underlying lesion can be seen reliably on plain radiographs and up to 41% of malignant vertebral lesions fail to show on plain X-rays of the spine. In cases of spinal infection, the plain X-ray can appear normal for up to eight weeks into the disease process (Bogduk & McGuirk 2002). A 'negative' or 'normal' X-ray does not, therefore, exclude underlying serious pathology of the spine and apparently normal radiographs could potentially mislead and be inappropriately reassuring.

However, plain radiographs show the greatest contrast with respect to bony structures and the tissues immediately surrounding them and so, if the cause of pain is suspected to be predominantly within the bone, a plain X-ray might help. A plain radiograph can be helpful in detecting:

- Osteomyelitis
- Discitis
- Paraspinal infections
- Tumours
- Fractures

Bogduk & McGuirk (2002) suggest that plain X-rays to detect serious pathology of the spine should be limited to those with:

- Previous cancer
- History of trauma

- Minor trauma in older patients
- Failure to respond to treatment

Most cases of adult mechanical low back pain should not be investigated with plain radiographs. Indeed, in line with current national guidance, most radiology departments will refuse to perform them unless there is a clear indication to do so. In this context, the criterion of 'failure to respond to treatment' must not be misused. The evidence tells us that the preferred treatment for the majority of cases presenting with simple mechanical low back pain should be an active rehabilitation programme. The question that has to be asked is whether the perceived failed treatment was actually evidence based. Some bizarre cases of non-evidence-based treatment will present to the clinician and should not be misinterpreted as failed treatment. We have come across cases where fillings in teeth have been removed as a consequence of the misconception that the amalgam used to fill teeth could cause back pain. Clearly, failure to respond to this 'treatment' is not surprising.

COMPUTED TOMOGRAPHY

Tomography, or imaging by sections, had been one of the pillars of radiologic diagnostics until the late 1970s. CT is a modification of the plain radiography technique and is used to produce a three-dimensional image. The scanner consists of a number of X-ray sources arranged on a rotating ring opposite corresponding digital detectors. As the ring is revolved around the patient, the beams are absorbed by the body tissues to varying degrees which the computer software can then reassemble into images representing three-dimensional slices through the body. Older scanners simply took multiple sequential image slices through the body to demonstrate the structures but the more modern spiral CT scanners corkscrew their way along the body and can obtain image data for a whole volume of body tissue very rapidly. Powerful computers allow these data to be reformatted in various planes or even as a three-dimensional image of structures, although the highest resolution images will always be in the same plane as the scanning unit. For spinal imaging, the most detailed images will always be in the transverse or axial plane.

CT scanning is considered to be a moderate to high radiation diagnostic technique and subjects patients to high levels of ionizing radiation. The effects of the radiation dose absorbed are cumulative over time and therefore repeated CT scans carry a higher risk of induced malignancy. It is therefore essential to avoid unnecessary repeated use of CT scans for an individual patient. Modern digital scanners use much lower radiation levels but the radiation dose is always significantly higher than that of plain radiographs. Typical lumbar spine CT scans expose the patient to 50 times the radiation of a chest X-ray and are therefore frequently localized to just a few spinal levels. It is therefore essential to give clear information on the radiology request card as to the exact clinical problem, otherwise the wrong region of the spine could be scanned, thus missing the pathology being considered.

CT scanning completely eliminates the degrading effects of the superimposition of images of structures outside the area of interest. In addition, the high contrast resolution of CT enables tissues that differ in physical density by less than 1% to be distinguished from each other. The resolution of CT scanning can be further enhanced by using contrast media, most frequently based on iodine compounds. These can be injected intravenously, or into body cavities or spaces such as joints or the spinal canal. Unfortunately, the relatively high incidence of allergic reactions to these contrast media can limit their use (Wikipedia 2006). Because X-ray techniques are particularly good at imaging bone tissue, CT scanning can be superior to MR scanning when looking for bone destruction or pathological fractures in the spine. However, because CT scanning is less able to resolve soft tissues than MR scanning, has less capability to be reformatted in multiple planes, and carries significant radiation risk when scanning large sections of the spinal column, it has largely been superseded by MR in investigating serious spinal pathology. It is not uncommon though to undertake high-resolution CT scans through specific areas of interest identified by MR scanning or plain radiographs.

MAGNETIC RESONANCE IMAGING (MR SCANNING)

MR scanning has now become the investigation of choice for most cases of spinal pathology and is particularly sensitive and specific at identifying serious spinal pathology. The technique involves the use of a carefully controlled but powerful magnetic field that causes the tissue molecules, especially the hydrogen ions in water molecules, to 'vibrate' or 'spin'. As the molecules are polarized by an electromagnetic pulse within the powerful magnetic field, they absorb energy, and when the magnetic field is relaxed, that energy is released as radio-frequency energy. The scanner detects this released radio-frequency energy and uses powerful computing techniques to reconstruct the signals into images.

MR scanning has many advantages. Images can be acquired in almost any plane. In the spine, the two most common imaging planes are sagittal and transverse, or axial. The exact plane of these images can be fine tuned to correct for positioning of the patient and to compensate for spinal deformities, such as scoliosis, and the axial images can be acquired in an inclined plane that correlates precisely with the individual intervertebral discs, thus compensating for any lordosis or kyphosis. Sometimes, frontal or coronal plane images are acquired and, indeed, images in almost any oblique plane can be requested depending on the indications.

Furthermore, by altering the timing of the energizing and relaxing phases of the cycle along with other characteristics of the electromagnetic field, different tissue types and characteristics can be demonstrated. The two most commonly used MR scanning sequences are 'T1-weighted' and 'T2-weighted'. In the broadest terms, T1-weighted images tend to demonstrate anatomical detail and T2-weighted images tend to demonstrate pathological features, although careful correlation of both sets of images is required to build a full picture of the clinical problem. Some scanning units clearly mark each sequence as T1 or T2, but where this annotation is missing, the sequence can be determined by comparison of the timing data imprinted on the image sections. A good rule of thumb is to assume that those images with fine detail and a broad range of grey scales are T1-weighted and those images that are coarser and of higher contrast are T2-weighted. Additional features are that fat shows with a high (bright) signal on T1-weighted images and water shows with a high signal on T2-weighted images. In the spine, the T2-weighted images will clearly demonstrate the CSF as a high signal column containing the darker spinal cord or nerve roots and will resemble the myelogram radiographs of former years. An additional way of remembering this is T2 = H_2O.

Occasionally, additional short T1 inversion recovery (STIR) sequences will be obtained. These are designed to suppress the signals generated by fat tissue, including fat in bone marrow. In the spine, these are often used to look for tumours and joint pathology, such as sacroileitis. It is also possible to enhance MR scans using gadolinium, an inert substance, usually injected intravenously for the purpose of enhancing vascular tissue. This can help to differentiate between a recurrent disc prolapse and post-operative inflammatory tissue following discectomy.

The strong magnetic field strengths and pulsing electromagnetic fields make MR scanning a contraindication in most patients with implanted or other metalic electronic medical devices, such as:

- Pacemakers
- Cochlear implants
- Insulin pumps
- Hydrocephalus shunts
- Neuro-stimulators
- Certain types of prosthetic heart valves and vascular stents

It is therefore essential to inform the radiology department in such cases, such as the type of implant, so that its MR compatibility can be checked. Ferrous metal implants, such as stainless steel fracture fixation plates or athroplasty components, can also be affected by the magnetic fields, although it is usually safe to scan such patients if the implant is well embedded and has been in place for several months. These implants can also cause large artefacts on the scan images. Titanium implants are less susceptible to these effects and are therefore preferentially used in spinal procedures. Small metal fragments in the eye, often the result of engineering activities such as welding or grinding without eye protection, can be moved or spun in the electromagnetic field and could cause severe damage and so it is common for orbital X-rays to be performed prior to MR scans in patients considered at risk.

MR scanning is an excellent modality to use if investigating soft tissue and is therefore ideal for imaging spinal structures. It is used frequently when neoplasm, infection or haemorrhage are suspected, as the following characteristically appear dark on T1-weighted images and light on T2 (Miller 2004):

- Water (including oedema)
- CSF
- Acute haemorrhage
- Soft tissue tumours

MR scanning is a valuable imaging technique in patients who are suspected of suffering from malignant spinal cord compression (MSCC). These patients (and those with suspected cauda equina compression) should have MR scans of the whole spine within 24 hours unless MR scanning is contraindicated. This should be done in time to allow definitive treatment to be planned and the integrity of the spinal cord protected.

The MR scan performed, at the radiologist's discretion, is likely to include sagittal T1 or STIR sequences of the whole spine, to prove or exclude the presence of spinal metastatic disease. Sagittal T2-weighted sequences may also be performed to identify the level and degree of compression of the spinal cord or cauda equina and to detect pathology within the cord itself. For patients with suspected MSCC or cauda equina syndrome in whom MR scanning is contraindicated, CT scanning may be the imaging modality of choice. However, if MSCC is suspected, urgent specialist opinion and advice are required and time should not be wasted struggling to arrange complex imaging (National Institute for Health and Clinical Excellence (NICE) 2008).

RADIO-ISOTOPE BONE SCAN

Radio-isotope bone scanning is primarily to detect bone abnormalities although under certain circumstances it can also show areas of increased blood flow that can occur at sites of infection and other disorders. The technique involves intravenous injection of a small volume of radioactive tracer attached to a bone substrate, usually technitium-99 methyl diphosphonate (MDP), which is then taken up by bone during new bone formation. The tracer emits γ rays, which are detected by the scanning device, known as a gamma camera. In a standard single phase bone scan, the patient is scanned two to four hours after the injection, by which time the isotope has been taken up by the osteoblasts and incorporated into the new bone matrix. The bone scan thus is a representation of osteoblastic activity. The normal skeleton, being constantly metabolically active, will therefore show a relatively uniform level of background activity. Any areas where new bone formation is increased will show up as areas of increased isotope activity or 'hot spots'. Conversely, any areas where new bone formation has ceased, such as in avascular necrosis, will show cold spots or 'photopenic' areas. Photopenic areas can also occur around tumours that inhibit osteoblastic activity (typically plasmacytoma or myeloma) and where bone destruction is so rapid that bone repair has no time to catch up (some aggressive osteolytic metastases). The pattern and exact location of these hot and cold spots will generally indicate the probable cause of the abnormality.

Bone scanning is extremely sensitive and will detect many abnormalities long before they can be seen on X-rays. Increased activity around stress and pathological fractures, for example, can be seen within 24 hours of injury, whereas it might take days or weeks for X-ray changes to become apparent. However, bone scanning is not very specific and often further investigations, such as X-rays or CT scans, of the abnormal areas are required to confirm the likely cause.

A modification of the standard bone scanning technique, known as a 'three-phase' scan, can be used to assess blood flow in a region of interest. This can be of greatest value in cases where infection is being considered (Bogduk & McGuirk 2002). Immediately after injection, the radio-isotope travels around the body in the arteries and then the veins. If a scan is taken immediately after injection, it will show the volume of blood flowing through the region being scanned. After a few minutes, the isotope diffuses from the vessels into the extracellular space, and this process will be faster at sites of inflammation or infection where the blow flow has increased and the capillaries have become more porous in response to the inflammatory process. Further scans taken 5–20 minutes after injection can thus show areas of increased activity around sites of infection.

The commonest reason for requesting an isotope bone scan will be to identify possible bone tumours or metastases. As the tumour destroys the surrounding bone, osteoblastic activity will increase in an attempt to repair the damage and this will show as a 'hot spot' at the site of the lesion. In cases of bone metastases, it is likely that there will be multiple hot spots scattered around the skeleton, typically in the ribs, vertebral bodies, pelvis, skull, proximal femur and proximal humerus. Occasionally, the bone destruction is so rapid, as in some forms of aggressive, osteolytic breast metastases, that the osteoblasts are destroyed before they have a chance to react and this might result in a false-negative result. Similarly, in myeloma the osteoblasts are probably inhibited by a tissue mediator produced by the tumour and the tumour lesions will therefore fail to show up on a bone scan until the surrounding bone becomes sufficiently weak to cause a pathological fracture (Miller 2004). Bone scanning is thus of little value in these situations and other investigations, such as blood tests and MR scanning, should be considered instead.

Radio-isotope bone scans are also very sensitive at detecting fractures, including stress fractures, and will often indicate increased activity around the fracture within hours before anything is evident on X-ray. This can be useful in detecting pars fractures and other stress lesions as well as osteoporotic vertebral collapse or other pathological fractures. It is often necessary to correlate these findings with plain radiographs to differentiate these reactive changes from degenerative change around the disc and facet joints.

DUAL ENERGY X-RAY ABSORPTIOMETRY (DEXA OR DXA)

DEXA scanning is a means of measuring bone mineral density (BMD), a measure of the mineral content (mainly calcium) contained in a certain volume of bone. This test is very reliable and is the gold standard of BMD measurement. A DEXA scan uses two low energy X-ray sources of different energies that are transmitted through the bone being tested. Computation subtracts the effects of soft tissue absorption leaving an accurate measurement of the absorption effect of the bone.

DEXA is mainly used to diagnose osteoporosis and risk of fracture. A statistical analysis is used to predict the likelihood of the patient either being osteoporotic or developing osteoporosis and thus gives a risk of fractures. The T-score is a comparison of a patient's BMD to that of a healthy 30-year-old of the same sex and ethnicity. The Z-score is the BMD corrected for the patient's age. A T-score of −2.5 or less is indicative of osteoporosis. This value is used in post-menopausal women and can also be used in men over aged 50 years. The thresholds for osteoporosis and osteopenia as described by the World Health Organization are (Wikipedia 2006):

- Osteoporosis – T-score of −2.5 or lower, i.e. bone density is 2.5 SD below the mean of a 30-year-old woman
- Osteopenia – T-score of less than −1.0 and greater than −2.5
- Normal – T-score of −1.0 or higher

A DEXA scan should be considered for (International Osteoporosis Foundation 2008; Wikipedia 2008):

- Women who have had a menopause or hysterectomy with ovaries removed before the age of 45 years.

- Women who have had a history of missed menstrual periods for reasons other than pregnancy, e.g. anorexia nervosa for a period of more than one year.
- Men with low testosterone levels.
- Men and women suffering from other conditions known to lead to bone loss, such as malabsorption syndrome, hyperparathyroidism and prolonged immobilization.
- Patients with a family history of maternal hip fracture <75 years of age.

References

Asher R 1954 Straight and crooked thinking. BMJ 2: 460–462

Binns A, Gurney H 1998 Update on hypercalcaemia in malignancy. Online. Available: www.medicineau.net.au (accessed 22 May 2006)

Bogduk N, McGuirk B 2002 Medical management of acute and chronic low back pain: an evidence based approach. Elsevier, Amsterdam

Cancer Research UK 2006 High calcium in people with cancer. Online. Available: www.cancerhelp.org.uk (accessed 22 May 2006)

Hicks M 2009 Research methods for clinical therapists, 5th edn. Churchill Livingstone, Elsevier, Edinburgh

International Osteoporosis Foundation 2008 Osteoporosis. Online. Available: www.iofbonehealth.org/home.html (accessed 2 July 2008)

Kochhar S, Marshall W 2003 Investigations: essential clinical chemistry. Student BMJ 11: 314–316

Kumar P, Clark M 2005 Clinical medicine, 6th edn. W B Saunders, Edinburgh

Lab Tests Online 2005 Online. Available: www.labtestsonline.org (accessed 6 July 2006)

Levack P, Graham J, Collie D et al 2002 Don't wait for a sensory level – listen to the symptoms: a prospective audit of the delays in diagnosis of malignant cord compression. Clinical Oncology 14: 472–480

McArdle W D, Katch F I, Katch V L 1991 Exercise physiology: energy, nutrition and human performance, 3rd edn. Lea & Febiger, Philadelphia

McGhee M 2005 A guide to laboratory investigations, 4th edn. Radcliffe Medical Press, Oxford

Medline Plus 2005 Hypercalcaemia. Online. Available: www. nlm.nih.gov/medlineplus

Miller M D 2004 Review of orthopaedics, 4th edn. W B Saunders, Philadelphia

National Institute for Health and Clinical Excellence 2008 Metastatic spinal cord compression: diagnosis and management of adults at risk of and with metastatic spinal cord compression. Clinical guideline 75. Online. Available: www.nice.org.uk/Guidance/CG75 (accessed 3 February 2009)

Net Doctor 2008 Multiple myeloma. Online. Available: www. netdoctor.co.uk/diseases/facts/multiplemyeloma.htm (accessed 18 July 2008)

Oken M M 2002 Management of myeloma: current and future approaches. Online. Available: www.moffitt.org/ moffittapps/ccj/v5n3/article2.html

Prostate Cancer Research Foundation 2008 Prostate cancer. Online. Available: www.thepcrf.org (accessed 9 July 2008)

Souhami R, Tobias J 1995 Cancer and its management, 2nd edn. Blackwell, Oxford

Squire C 2003 Laboratory handbook. Morecambe Bay Hospitals NHS Trust, Lancaster

Wikipedia 2006 Online. Available: http://en.wikipedia.org (accessed 5 July 2006)

Index

NB: Page numbers in **bold** refer to figures and tables

Printed in the United States
By Bookmasters